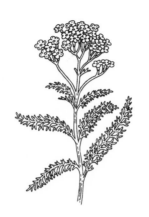

NATURALLY INSPIRED

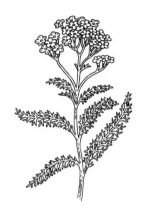

NATURALLY INSPIRED

Natural lifestyle practices and remedies
to boost immunity in children and families.

Written By
Meghan Rose | Elaine Shtein | Kimberly Koebensky
Dr. Troy Jaques | K.J. Moore, RN, BSN | Elizabeth Goebel
Melissa Weber | Suzzie Vehrs, B.S. | Carrie Lee
Jennifer Schmid, MSN, RN, CNL, PHN, ACN | Brittany Love
Noemi Elizabeth Hermling | Laira De La Vega
Julie A. Miller, B.S.; A.C.N. | Lesa Ritchie Craig, HHC

Published in Canada, for Global Distribution by Golden Brick Road Publishing House Inc.

www.goldenbrickroad.pub
For more information email: kylee@gbrph.ca

ISBN:
Paperback: 978-1-988736-69-3

To order additional copies of this book: orders@gbrph.ca

CONTENTS

INTRODUCTION

By Meghan Rose

From the time I was a little girl, I have known that I wanted to have a career in which I was truly helping people, so it was fitting for me to end up in the field of nursing. I started my career working in infectious diseases, later moving into elementary school nursing and finally orthopedics before I retired to stay home with my young children. My experiences as a nurse were profound, and I am forever grateful for this path that I wound up on. I learned a lot more than I had ever imagined.

Some significant takeaways from my time in the medical field include:

- There are a lot of people who need medical help.
- Medicine is a business . . . a business that profits from sick people.
- Medicine is also political. There is a money trail to be followed among government agencies, politicians, pharmaceutical companies, and medical establishments.
- Conventional Western medicine operates mostly through the prescription of pharmaceutical drugs, which come with a laundry list of side effects, some worse than the actual disease the prescription is meant to treat.
- Pharmaceuticals never address the root cause of an issue. They are a bandage to cover up and manage symptoms.
- Advances in healthcare logically should mean that we see *fewer* specialty clinics popping up; instead we see more. More urgent care centers, more childhood cancer centers, more dialysis clinics, more imaging centers, more Alzheimer's care centers . . . you get the picture.
- Despite being so medically "advanced," the United States has a higher infant and childhood mortality rate than many other industrialized nations.[1]

- According IQVia (formerly IMS Health), a company that provides information, services, and technology for the healthcare industry, 7,213,599 children between the ages of zero and seventeen are on some form of psychiatric medication.[2]

And yet, despite how disturbing this looks when it's put on paper, all of these things are now accepted as a normal part of childhood and a way of life.

Whereas when I grew up, I did not know a single person with autism, ADHD, speech impediments, or *any* other neurological disorder or chronic illness . . . now we have entire classrooms dedicated to children with special needs. Food allergies, learning disabilities, and neurological disorders such as autism and epilepsy are on the rise, as are juvenile diabetes, childhood cancer, ADHD, and other disorders.

This way of life may be common, but there is absolutely *nothing* normal about it.

For most of my life, I thought holistic health was quackery . . . until through my own experience with my son's ADHD and subsequent frightening reactions to his medication for it, I found that true health transformation can only happen through holistic means. It is the only way to address the root cause of the development of an environmentally triggered condition.

Parents have so much conflicting information to sift through that it can seem overwhelming. I believe the medical industry absolutely has its place, and my goal in writing this book is not to shame anybody. Rather, I want to present factual information that will inspire people to do their *own* research into everything, in turn empowering them to make choices that they are one hundred percent confident in because they know *why* they are making them. My goal is to inspire parents to dig deeper into learning how the body functions holistically and to let them know that there is hope in what can seem like a scary world where chronic disease is rampant.

My hope is that by educating and empowering one person at a time, we can take back our children's health and create a better future for all of them.

01

KNOW BETTER, DO BETTER

By Elaine Shtein

"I own and embrace the negative inner emotions that aren't serving me, breathe and release them, and move on. I am so proud of the person I have become."

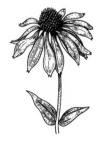

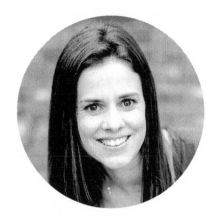

Elaine knew from a young age that she wanted to be a teacher. She earned a bachelor's degree in psychology from the University of California at San Diego and completed a master's degree in bilingual education (Spanish) from the University of California at Davis. After spending twelve years teaching kindergarten and first, second, and third grade, she retired to spend more time with her family. When Elaine's son was diagnosed with autism, it acted as a wake-up call to research information for herself. As Elaine learned more about how to help her son, and about the underlying causes that led to his diagnosis, she found her passion and voice. She now shares her story and advocates for parents with special needs children. She also works with families to reduce their household toxicity. Elaine truly believes that it is possible to be healthy and thrive in today's world but that doing so takes knowing where to find reliable information. Elaine now works from home as a partner with Hempworx, the fastest growing online CBD company. Elaine lives in San Jose, CA with her husband, Misha, their daughter, Sophia, and their son, Jackson.

www.elaineshtein.com
ig: @elaineshtein | fb: @eshtein

P eople say I have a familiar face. It's like they know me from somewhere, like they've met me before, like I have a familiar energy. Maybe it is my welcoming, nurturing demeanor. I am not superior or inferior to anyone. I am doing the best I can with what I know. I am not a doctor, a pharmacist, a nurse, or a scientist. I am a mother, woman, friend, citizen.

I was called to be a mother. Welcoming my two beautiful babies, Sophia and Jackson, into my life shifted my world; they completed me. I was *that* mom who went to all the baby classes and researched the best car seats, cribs, and jogger strollers. I had the nursery ready for months before the babies were born. I was active in the online mommy communities, connecting with fellow moms — new, veteran, and expectant. I read the magazines and the parenting books and listened to every piece of advice my midwife gave to ensure I was up to date with all the latest tips and tricks to be the best possible mother.

As mothers, we know every freckle, every giggle, every cry and the slightest whimper. We know when our babies need to be burped, snuggled, tickled, and fed. It's our mama bear instinct to protect our children, provide everything we can for them, and do what's best for them — to give them every opportunity to fully thrive.

I live by Maya Angelou's words: *"I did then what I knew how to do. Now that I know better, I do better."*[3] I believe that people are doing the best they can with what they know. When my children were born, I didn't know what I know now. But I am committed to always learning, growing, and evolving. Science is never settled; credible new studies are always forthcoming. The day we become set in our ways and closed to new ideas and information is a sad, scary day. Jackson's diagnosis was a slap in the face, my wake-up call to the fact that I had not been presented with the information I deserved to make the best medical choices for my child.

I share Jackson's story with you out of love and truth and with an open heart because it deserves to be shared. As loving mothers, fathers, and citizens, we deserve to be fully informed to make the best choices for our children, for all children. What I have learned in nearly a decade of research has changed my entire outlook and my daily choices for my family's health.

After spending thousands of hours conducting research online, attending conferences, reading books, watching documentaries, and experiencing first-hand Jackson's spiral into severe autism, I know better. I know so much better. My eyes are open; I am wide awake, I found my voice, and I am committed to sharing Jackson's story and our journey so that others can avoid the hardships, heartache, and stresses that come with a child with severe, non-verbal autism. Learn from me.

As you read my story, I ask that you not judge. I was doing the best with what I knew. This is my story — raw, real, and unfiltered. Whatever stage you are at in your path of awareness, research, and learning, I hope that this chapter and book help you along your journey to healing yourself, your child, or whatever else needs healing in your life and that you pay it forward and share it with someone else.

Sophia, my firstborn, was born in 2007. Motherhood didn't disappoint; I was indeed a natural, juggling all facets of my life and loving it! I was teaching first grade, taking Sophia to daycare, playing ponies and princesses, taking family outings on the weekend, and enjoying experiencing Sophia's development. She was such a joy: a happy, curious, adventurous baby who loved exploring new things. Sophia kept hitting all her milestones, and her strong, loving, playful personality reaffirmed our desire to have a second child.

Enter Jackson. On May 26, 2009, I was thirty-eight weeks pregnant with our baby boy. After a routine check-up, my midwife called to say my blood pressure was elevated. She recommended I go directly to the hospital to be induced. Heavy doses of Pitocin, an epidural, and six pushes later, my husband and I tearfully welcomed our beautiful, precious, perfect baby boy, Jackson. Our family was complete, now a family of four.

Jackson was vaccinated from day one, according to the CDC's recommended schedule. Once again, I was that perfect mom scheduling the "well baby" visits, always happy to see that Jackson was progressing and growing, in the ninetieth percentile for height and weight. I nursed Jackson from the start. He was a good eater, a peaceful sleeper, a playful peek-a boo-er, and an adventurous crawler and then walker. He developed typically that first year and was just as explorative, curious, and happy as Sophia, keeping up with his older sister.

After Jackson's one-year pediatrician visit, we noticed some changes in his behavior and health. In one single visit, he received ten doses of seven vaccines (hepatitis B, rotavirus, DPT, flu, pneumococcal, MMR, and polio). He weighed twenty-four pounds; looking back, it was an alarmingly high dose of many viruses at once to receive at only one year of age, when his immune system was still developing. By that time, I had stopped nursing and had been feeding him a soy-based formula for a few months. Additionally, we had a gardener who was spraying commercial pesticides outside our home to keep the critters away. To top it off, I was adding fluoride drops to the kids' water and buying conventional produce and foods from the supermarket.

I didn't know. After all, this is what we all do, right? We do the best we can with all that we have, all that we are aware of in any present moment. I didn't know the detrimental effects that all the abovementioned practices could have on my sweet boy's health.

I trusted our pediatrician and her seven-plus years of extensive, specialized education. I trusted her when she gave me that prescription for fluoride drops. Of course, I didn't want my babies to be in pain when they got their shots, so I gave them liquid pain reliever before and after. Let's face it — we are not always presented with all the facts we need to make the best possible decisions in the name of health.

I didn't know.

By the time Jackson was fifteen months old, we knew something was seriously wrong. For several months, he had not been his typical self. He stopped playing peek-a-boo, self-limited his food choices, and only wanted to drink milk. He was content to sit by himself and flip through the same book for extended periods of time. He had rigid self-soothing behaviors, such as holding the same two alphabet letters in his hands, sprinkling rocks, and spinning anything circular.

I remember one particular morning so clearly. Jackson was in his high chair, drinking his milk and watching the movie *Cars* with his sister. He was in a daze, a zone, not laughing at the parts Sophia was laughing at, not reacting to our dog licking his feet. He was in his own world, a world far away. Something wasn't right. I walked over, stood behind him, and said, "Jackson!" in a high-pitched, fun mom-voice. No response. I said his name again, this time a little louder.

"Jackson!"

No response. I moved to the left, got really close, and sang his name in an even more fun and engaging voice.

"Jackson!"

Nothing, not even a flinch or a head turn.

Assuming he was hard of hearing, my husband and I took Jackson to an audiologist. He passed the hearing tests but was still in his own world, neither happy nor sad. Just flat, lifeless, and zoned out.

We scheduled an appointment with our pediatrician. She read fifteen questions from a checklist and recorded our answers. By the end of that visit, after seeing Jackson spinning, rocking, and flapping, she gave us the requisition to go to our local regional center for an official autism diagnosis so we could start getting services for early intervention. By the age of eighteen months, Jackson was officially diagnosed with severe autism. He started an intensive forty hours a week of applied behavioral analysis (ABA) therapy, speech therapy, and occupational therapy.

We were officially thrown into the world of autism, with no manual, no guidance; our world flipped upside down. As I researched how best to address the underlying body disregulation that contributed to Jackson's autism, we tried many behavioral and medical interventions: twenty-four-hour EEG, gluten-free/dairy-free/organic diet, hyperbaric oxygen chamber, antifungals, antivirals, methylated B-12 shots, parasite treatment, homotoxicology, osteopathy, craniosacral therapy, Son-Rise playroom, CBD oil, oral chelation, glutathione IV, mitochondrial supplements, stem cells in Panama, homeopathy, chiropractic, reiki, essential oils, bone broth, IonCleanse footbath, GcMAF probiotic yogurt, Rapid Prompting Method,

Biomat, and various MAPS (Medical Academy of Pediatrics Special Needs) doctors for customized supplement plans.

We spent tens of thousands of dollars out of pocket on these doctors, specialists, and interventions. Going into the specifics of each of these interventions would require an entire book of my own. What I know for sure is one case of autism is one case of autism — what works for one child may not for another. I don't regret any of the interventions we've tried, since each one provided information about Jackson's underlying body disregulation. We still use many of them today because they are a foundation for optimal health.

If I found a magic lantern and had a genie grant me three wishes, I would only ask for one: to know then what I know now. To know about the corrupt vaccine industry, the toxic GMO food, and the unresearched cumulative effects of these toxins. My research began at the CDC website, looking up the ingredients in vaccines. Aluminum, formaldehyde, Polysorbate 80, aborted fetal tissue, monkey kidney cells, egg proteins??[4] I researched each ingredient's individual health outcomes and looked for the studies showing that these ingredients in combined doses were safe and healthy and well-researched. Those studies don't exist. I was shocked, as if I had been punched in the gut and had the wind knocked out of me. Next I looked at a vaccine package insert, that folded-up paper in the box with the vaccine vial that lists all the adverse reactions, contraindications, and important information specific to each vaccine.[5] Then I learned about the National Childhood Vaccine Injury Act (NCVIA), a law passed in the U.S. in 1986 under the Reagan Administration. This law waived all liability from vaccine manufacturers, thus preventing people from being able to take legal action against them.[6] I do not attribute Jackson's autism to vaccines alone. My vaccine research spilled into other areas of toxic exposure. I wasn't prepared for what I learned:

- There are 84,000 industrial chemicals used in household items.[7]
- The FDA has tested two hundred chemicals.[8]
- The FDA regulates five chemicals.[9]

I finally understood the fact that governmental agencies don't have our health as a priority, that just because something is on a store shelf doesn't mean it has been tested or is safe. I delved into the toxicity of our food supply, cleaning and personal care products, and water supply and the unresearched short- and long-term outcomes of this massive chemical exposure.[10] My biggest takeaway after thousands of hours delving deep: for my family to be happy, healthy and thriving, I had to research for myself.

What's done is done. There are no do-overs after vaccinating. I made uninformed choices and now must live with them. Jackson has round-the-clock needs; he is non-verbal and unaware of danger and will require constant care. That being said, not a day goes by when I don't believe unwaveringly that Jackson will speak, learn self-care skills, and heal to the point where he can be the best, most independent version of himself. Autism is medical, and as we address the components keeping our kids inflamed and toxic, their health continues to improve. So where do I go from here? I will never give up on Jackson and his potential. We will continue to travel to see specialists, put in the time to research new interventions and medical advances, and love him every day.

I experienced every emotion imaginable after Jackson's diagnosis: guilt, shame, fear, overwhelm, resentment, self-blaming, depression, anxiety, and doubt. I lived in these negative, low-vibrational energies for the first few years of our new life with autism. I want to be transparent and keep it real — it was tough. My once-perfect baby now faced major challenges. His life was forever changed; our family's life was forever changed. I blamed myself. Those were some dark years, with a lot of crying and sifting through emotions, but I still had to pull myself together enough to be a mom, researcher, supplement prepper, teacher, wife, and cook. I felt so alone, isolated, like the only mom of a child with autism. I felt like nobody else could possibly understand what our family was going through.

These years wreaked havoc on my own health. I was in a fight-or-flight state for many years, putting myself last and taking care of everyone else's needs and health but my own. I was gaining weight, experiencing massive brain fog and low energy; eventually, I faced the diagnosis of thyroid cancer at age thirty-five. My mindset, food choices, and lifestyle were toxic. They were killing me softly.

So what changed? How did I go from this low-vibration, toxic mindset to an empowered, loving, knowing mindset?

I made a choice, first about the people I surrounded myself with. I started finding my autism community and seeing children and moms thriving despite hardships. Then I started scheduling in my own self-care. Reading books that inspired me. Working out, getting in nature, moving my body. Preparing nourishing, healing foods for myself. Avoiding toxic chemicals. Hiring a coach to ask me the tough questions, allowing me the space to be vulnerable and heal the negative emotions that were keeping me stuck. Researching the toxic agenda until I felt like a self-proclaimed expert, knowledgeable and able to guide others in their research.

My shift in energy continues to be a daily commitment and practice, a gift to myself. No matter what unknown, unpredictable chaos comes our way from the tornado of autism, I have equipped myself with the tools, mindset, and stamina to get through it. I have the inner knowing that negative emotions can't be a long-term part of my core belief system if I want to live a full life of love, abundance, and truth. I own and embrace the negative inner emotions that aren't serving me, breathe and release them, and move on. I am so proud of the person I have become.

As Jackson continues to grow, new and unforeseen challenges appear daily. I know that there will always be something unknown or unexpected that can happen in our lives. I also know that amidst the chaos that is life, the only constant is me — my response to situations, my mindset, my ability to constantly find ways to be better, to do better, to live better. The power lies within me.

02

A CHILD IN A TOXIC WORLD

By Kimberly Koebensky

"I speak from experience here that
a worried mother will do better research
than the FBI."

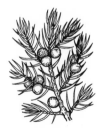

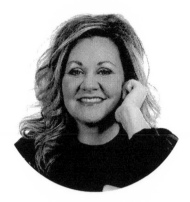

Kimberly Koebensky is a former corporate slave (ranging from top recruiter in the nation to top outside sales producer with previous employers) turned passionate and driven entrepreneur. She is now a multi-six-figure earner and top leader in a Global Wellness company, building her business right from home.

Kimberly lives in a small town in Northern Minnesota with her two beautiful boys and is happily married to her husband, Brody. She is intensely passionate about her faith, as well as about educating people to make safer choices in nutrition, personal care, and cleaning products and to reduce their overall toxic body burden. After falling ill in 2009 and spending seven years battling multiple health challenges, she took her health into her own hands and became a self-advocate.

In May 2016, Kimberly discovered Nutrigenomic products, which not only changed but actually saved her life in a short five days. She now takes pride in helping others use Nutrigenomic products to support their body's natural cellular function and upregulate their genes' ability to produce their own God-given antioxidants. She loves anything holistic and organic and wants nothing more than to inspire families to improve their physical and financial health and live better lives.

www.KimberlyK.info
fb: kimberly harvey koebensky

"He who has health, has hope, and he who has hope has everything."
~ Arabian proverb

May 2009 — a time I will never forget. I was planning my wedding to the man of my dreams when I suddenly fell ill. Over the previous few years, I had gone through several stressful life events that had a profound effect on my health, so it was no surprise I ended up getting sick. One day I was fine; the next I was going through intense testing for multiple sclerosis (MS) after doctors diagnosed me with optic neuritis. Thankfully, I was not diagnosed with MS, but never in a million years did I think I was about to suffer years full of health difficulties: miscarriages, depression, anxiety, daily dizziness, and gut issues, to name just a few. It was an eye-opening experience for me and for everyone in my life.

My biggest dream, and that of my husband, was to start a family together. In September 2009, we got good news about my health — we could move forward with trying to conceive a baby. The thought of having a baby with someone who is the true love of my life was the best feeling I had ever experienced, other than the day my first son, Charlie (now fourteen), was born. Raising small humans was both thrilling and daunting, but I was *so* ready to embark on the journey of conceiving a second child.

That journey started with back-to-back miscarriages and then a two-year lull. I felt like a failure. *What was wrong with me?* We were full of heartache and wondered whether God had it in His plans for us to have a child. We endured many failed fertility treatments. *Why was my body not working?* When I finally had a complete blood panel done, it showed I was compound heterozygous for the MTHFR gene. My doctors all dismissed this finding as no big deal so we forged on. However, they now considered me a "high-risk" patient if I got pregnant because I was thirty-five years old. We kept trying and prayed so much.

On August 8, 2011, I found out I was pregnant with my son Keegan, who is now seven years old. Three days after Keegan was born, I experienced a pulmonary embolism that almost took my life. I dug deeper into MTHFR and realized that it is, in fact, a thing. Methylenetetrahydrofolate reductase deficiency, in a nutshell, means I have a significantly decreased ability to remove toxic chemicals from my body. I read multiple articles, and many of them kept pointing out the need for nontoxic, safe personal care and cleaning products. *What?* You mean to tell me that after all these years, I am just now finding out that my makeup, deodorant, perfume, lotion, laundry detergent, and cleaning products are full of toxic ingredients? It baffled me. All I could think about was that I recently had a child inside me. What did I just inadvertently do to him? How has he been affected?

I speak from experience here that a worried mother will do better research than the FBI. I became a label reader overnight, wanting to become an expert in everyday toxic exposure so I could inform and educate people on how to make better, safer choices. I looked at every label in our house, wrote down the names of the ingredients, and researched each one. I was in complete disbelief. Why would these chemicals knowingly be placed in our products? I went to my children's products. *Same thing.* I was sick to my stomach.

We can no longer take for granted that what we see on shelves in the store is healthy. Did you know that there are 84,000 chemicals registered in the United States,[11] only two hundred of which have been assessed for safety?[12] The last time they passed a federal law regulating cosmetics was in 1938; that means it has been over eighty years since Congress last updated the federal law to ensure that personal care products are safe![13] The Food and Drug Administration doesn't even require basic safety testing for ingredients in personal care products before someone uses them.[14] If that isn't scary enough, according to the Environmental Working Group (EWG), an average of two hundred industrial chemicals and pollutants can be found in babies' umbilical cord blood.[15] *Their lifeline!* Before a child even has the privilege of entering this world, they have been exposed to hundreds of toxic chemicals.

I have never been so inspired to be loud. To share with others this information I never knew existed. If a mom like me, who takes pride in doing the best job I can to provide the safest environment for my family, didn't know these facts, *many* others are in the same shoes. I want to protect my children and our family as much as I can. Our children aren't an informed group of people who have control over their environment. Unlike adults, they are both unaware of the risks and unable to make proper choices to protect their own health. They use what we provide for them. The more we can educate ourselves and others to make better choices, the more things will change in this world.

It might shock parents to know that companies are free to use almost any ingredient in children's personal care products. Some products may state they are "natural" yet use artificial preservatives. Others that claim to be "gentle" contain harsh skin irritants. These days, with such scant regulation and such clever marketing that greenwashes people, you almost have to become a detective to figure out what is healthy for your children. Potential risks from these chemicals can encompass anything from allergic reactions to hormone disruption, reproductive damage, cancer, and more.

Our skin is our largest organ and our first line of defense. It serves as protection against extreme temperatures and toxic chemicals; it also produces antibacterial compounds that ward off infection and is one of the six organs of detoxification, helping to usher out some of the toxins that end up inside of us. Our skin is permeable and can easily absorb much of what it touches; we know this because certain pharmaceuticals are delivered transdermally, such as birth control and the nicotine patch. These chemicals can build up in the body so it is crucial to limit our exposure. Children spend lots of time playing on the ground and putting things in their mouth. In addition, the amount of air they breathe, food they eat, and liquids they drink is larger for their size than it is for adults, so chemical levels can soar even if they are doing the same things we do. It is so crucial to be vigilant in your choices because children are not just little adults; they are still growing at a rapid pace, and there are windows of vulnerability in which their immune, neurological, reproductive, endocrine, digestive, and entire bodily development can be permanently damaged from environmental toxins and harsh chemicals. Studies show that even small chemical exposures during critical windows can lead to breast cancer, infertility, learning disabilities, and other serious problems later in life.[16]

There is good news, though. If you know what to look for and how to make safer choices by avoiding products with harmful chemicals, you can lower the toxin levels in your body almost immediately. Many of the ingredients used in today's personal care and cleaning products are difficult to pronounce; in addition, there are not just one or two but multiple toxic ingredients present in just a single product. A chemical cocktail is great way to describe some of these unsafe concoctions.

Some big offenders to look for include:

Flame retardants: These are found in children's pajamas, bedding, car seat covers, and foam baby products. Studies show that flame retardants immediately enter the bloodstream and urine; in addition, research has linked these chemicals to long-term impacts such as endocrine disruption, lower IQ, ADD, fertility issues, thyroid disease, and cancer.[17] What is even worse, studies show that these chemicals can't prevent fires and have been proven unnecessary.[18] Safer fabric choices include organic cotton, cotton, and wool.

Phthalates: These are a group of chemicals used to soften and increase flexibility in plastic and are largely found in scented cleaning and personal care products and food packaging. Think cartoon-branded generic body wash with the strong smell of fake fruit! People may think these products are "cute," but what isn't so cute is the damage that phthalates can cause. Phthalates are endocrine disruptors linked to increased allergic reactions, asthma, developmental disorders, decreased fertility, and even reproductive malformations in males. They've also been identified by Project TENDR (Targeting Environmental Neuro-Developmental Risks) "as a prime example of chemicals emerging concern to brain development."[19] The solution to reducing your exposure is to choose safe, organic, fragrance-free products and eliminate all use of plastic food storage containers.

Formaldehyde: This is a known human carcinogen and can be found in shampoo and bath products for babies and children. Formaldehyde is also often found in liquid soaps such as hand and body wash. However, even when products are contaminated with this chemical, you won't always see it on the label. While formaldehyde can be added directly to a product, it is also a toxic byproduct of chemical manufacturing and product formulation and can be released over time in small amounts from certain preservatives used in a product. It is anything but safe and has been linked to cancer and skin allergies.[20]

BPA and BPA substitutes: Think baby bottles, plastic Paw Patrol or Mickey Mouse plate and cup sets, any type of sippy cup, and other food storage or feeding containers. BPA could have multiple detrimental side effects such as neurological and immune disorders, increased risk for a wide range of cancers, and increased risk of obesity.[21] BPA can affect the entire body and is not recommended for children.[22] In 2012, the FDA banned BPA in baby bottles and children's sippy cups. The bad news is that the products they have been using to take the place of BPA (BPS, BPE, BPF, and many others) are just as unhealthy and toxic. Some studies suggest that almost *all* plastics have estrogenic activity and potentially leach endocrine-disrupting chemicals.[23] In our house now, we use glass and stainless steel containers for everything, including drinking bottles, food storage, and straws.

The world today is so different from what it used to be. I know my parents never knew about or worried about these issues when I was growing up. I have described just a few of the biggest toxic offenders, but there are so many more, from the chemicals in the furniture we sit and sleep on and the pharmaceutical drugs and antibiotics we are prescribed to the highly toxic ingredients in vaccines. Sugary juices and conventional pasteurized milk, the fluoride and triclosan in toothpaste, laundry chemicals, heavy metals and contaminants in our water supply, artificial dyes and flavors in food, chemicals in sunscreen . . . I think you get my point. We need to question everything today. It is tough to be a child in this toxic world.

It is easy for anyone to get overwhelmed and not know where to start. I felt the same way when this knowledge first came into my life, but I took it all day by day and started to replace one or two products at a time. There are so many affordable options out there today, and many people even make their own products. Reducing your chemical exposure can be a scary task when you are just starting out, so begin by reading labels. The packaging may be full of marketing terms such as "herbal," "natural," or "hypoallergenic." Manufacturers will make a lot of claims on their packaging because, quite frankly, they can. Don't be fooled by their creativity and attractive wording. To truly find out what is in your products, read the ingredients on the label and learn how to decipher them for safety. Research each one. The EWG's *Skin Deep* website search engine and *Healthy Living* smartphone app are a great place to start for that.

We vote with our dollars every single day. If we buy products time and time again, we create a demand for them. If we turn a deaf ear or a blind eye to what we hear and see, changes will never happen. I have done everything in my power to make a positive impact on people's lives; when I learn something new, I share it. People deserve to know this information and will welcome it with open arms once they find out its effects on their loved ones. Once you know better, I promise you will do better.

It infuriates me as a mom of two healthy boys that we have to go to such great lengths to keep them safe. In a perfect world, we would walk into a store, be able to grab anything off the shelves, and be at peace that it is safe and healthy for all of us. I have learned so much in the last several years and will continue to be a student. We must continue to advocate for our health and safety and for the sake of our children; no one else is going to do that for us. We as parents can make healthy choices overall by using fewer personal care products on our children. Know your environment. Protect your health. If we do not have our health, we have nothing.

03

ADJUSTING TO LIFE: SPECIFIC CHIROPRACTIC CARE

By Dr. Troy Jaques

"Life is always better when your head is on straight."

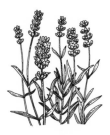

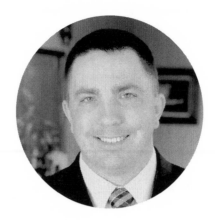

Troy Jaques studied at Life University in Marietta, Georgia. While he wanted to be a chiropractor from the beginning, he knew he did not want to be a rack-and-crack type of chiropractor. After his daughter had an unfortunate accident, he found his true passion for specific upper cervical chiropractic work.

Troy opened up his own office in Twin Falls, Idaho in 2014. His patients love the tagline that they "need to get their heads on straight." Nothing is more rewarding for Troy than seeing people get off their medications. He truly believes that what makes a great doctor is how many medications you can get a patient off rather than how many medications you put a person on.

The uniqueness of what Troy does has allowed him to create a special niche in his community for better healthcare. He is able to improve multiple ailments and illnesses to the point of non-existence and optimal health, something allopathic doctors only dream of doing better. He has successfully helped patients with Parkinson's disease, migraines, glaucoma, allergies, asthma, and sciatica, all by taking proper care of the upper cervical spine. He does not "treat" these conditions, but he recognizes that the entire body is under the control of the nervous system and that a properly functioning nervous system allows the body to heal.

www.tfuppercervical.com

My name is Dr. Troy Jaques, and I am a specific upper cervical chiropractor. If you do not know what that is, you are not alone. In simplest terms, it is a specialty within the field of chiropractic that deals directly with the brainstem, the area at the top part of the neck where the brain turns into the spinal cord.

The power that made the body can heal the body under the right circumstances. When the sperm and the egg come together, the first thing that is formed is the brainstem. From that point on, the nervous system controls the entire body. From the beginning, the brainstem dictates how the rest of the body will form. If a vertebra in the top of the neck becomes misaligned, it creates pressure and an unfavorable environment for the body to heal itself and return to a normal homeostatic state.

Before we get too far into this, you'll need to understand the human anatomy a bit more, specifically the spine. The spine is made up of five different sections. It starts with seven cervical vertebrae at the top. Next we have twelve thoracic vertebrae, the five lumbar vertebrae, and finally the sacrum and coccyx at the bottom."[24] The sacrum and coccyx form a solid piece; for our purposes here, we do not need to pay much attention to them. Here is what you do need to know: From the second cervical vertebra down, each vertebra has a bony lock system called transverse processes, in which the bones interlock via facet joints. This system makes it really difficult for that part of the spine to truly misalign. The top bone in the neck, on the other hand, is called the atlas and is completely different than the rest of the spine. This bone can misalign in three different directions. Chiropractors consider this to be a "sloppy joint" between the skull above and the second cervical vertebra (called the axis) below. This makes the top part of the spine the most vulnerable area of the entire spine.

Every nerve in the entire body travels through the brainstem. If the atlas becomes misaligned, then any part of the body can be compromised. Once chiropractors set the atlas in the correct position, we make every effort not to adjust it again. Every time a joint gets an adjustment of any kind, it weakens the tendons and ligaments, thus creating more of a problem. Healing the body comes from holding an adjustment, not simply from adjusting. The longer the atlas stays in place, the healthier the individual will become and the stronger the tendons and ligaments will get as time goes on. This is why chiropractors use specific thermal instrumentation to determine whether the bone is misaligned and x-rays to determine how to fix the misalignment without guesswork.

Common problems seen by upper cervical doctors include migraines, seizures, digestive problems, sleeping disorders, and sciatica. All these issues and so many more can be addressed by making sure the atlas is in the proper position.

The brain sends out signals telling your toes to wiggle, your heart to beat, and so forth. All those signals pass through the brainstem. However, if the atlas is misaligned and those signals cannot pass through correctly, what happens to them? The signals can become disrupted. I joke by saying we need to get the head on straight, but in reality, if the brain cannot communicate with the rest of the body at the optimal rate of one hundred percent, then the patient will have problems. Likewise, if the brain can communicate at one hundred percent capacity with the rest of the body, the body has an increased chance of healing itself naturally.

My daughter's story led me down the road to understanding what true health is. The two biggest lessons I learned are that health does not come from a needle and that structure determines function. If the spinal structure is not correct, the body will not function correctly either. I've discovered that this principle is something that allopathic means — i.e., a vaccine — could never compete with.

I grew up getting vaccinated. I believed vaccines were good. Looking back, my arguments in favor of vaccines were ridiculous. My belief caused contention in my marriage because my wife was against vaccines. However, I was very pushy and got my way to have my oldest daughter, Kate, vaccinated as a baby. Not a day goes by that I do not regret doing that. I regret vaccinating her because I did not do my own research. I did not do my due diligence to actually know what was best for my child. I left all of that up to the "experts." At the end of the day, it is my responsibility as the parent to take care of my children, not that of doctors, scientists, and the government. That was a failure on my part. I did not research how to heal ailments naturally. Through my later studies, however, I got hooked on learning all about vaccines and how toxic and poisonous they are. I discovered that while we could take care of our daughter's body structurally, if we injected her with vaccines she would still not be at optimal health.

When Kate was very young, she fell down a flight of stairs. Her atlas came out of place, putting abnormal pressure on her brainstem. This created a vagal nerve dysfunction. The vagus nerve is the tenth cranial nerve. It comes off the brainstem and controls the heart, lungs, stomach, abdomen, liver, pancreas, and intestines. Because the vagus nerve controlling her lungs was kinked, Kate began coughing a very dry, unproductive cough. I was getting ready to move to Atlanta, Georgia to go to chiropractic school when the accident happened. I knew I wanted to be a chiropractor so I tried doing everything I could to take care of the problem naturally. But after seeking out several different chiropractors and other holistic doctors to help my little girl, nothing was working. The chiropractors treated her the best they could, but their techniques were not taking the pressure off the brainstem. We then took her to a naturopathic doctor who gave her some herbs to settle her throat. Again, the root cause was neglected and the cough persisted. (Please do not think that these things never work; they do, just not in our case at the time.)

Kate's cough was getting worse. Every other breath was a cough. It literally changed how we lived. One Sunday, I would go to church while my wife stayed home with her; the next Sunday, we would switch roles. We finally sought out modern medical help. To this day, I still have no idea what kind of drugs they put Kate on, but they also proved to be of no use. One medical doctor said my three-year-old had been faking this cough for the past year.

At this point, I was frustrated enough with the doctors to listen to anyone who could get Kate better, or even *thought* they could get her better. A close friend of mine told me to take her to a specific upper cervical chiropractor. I had never heard of such a thing. He told me that every nerve in the body travels through the brainstem and that once the pressure was taken off Kate's brainstem, she would get better. At our wits' end, we took her to a specific upper cervical doctor. He made a specific correction to the atlas and immediately her symptoms began to dissipate. Healing takes time, but two months later, Kate's cough was gone.

That was almost ten years ago. I decided to put all my eggs in one basket and learned all I could about specific upper cervical chiropractic care. If a specific atlas correction could fix a cough, what else could it fix?

Specific upper cervical chiropractic care is based on making a very precise correction to the atlas or, in rare cases, to the second cervical vertebra called the axis. X-rays of the neck are taken to determine exactly how to make that correction. After the correction is made, the patient will rest on their back for about half an hour to hold the adjustment in place. When everything is done properly, patients require very little additional adjusting thereafter. Once the top of the neck has healed, seldom does any other body part need to be manipulated. For this reason, the brainstem can be dubbed the "Houston Control Center" of the body.

Do you remember Christopher Reeve? He was the actor who played Superman and suffered a fatal neck injury from a horseback riding accident in 1995. According to a study of the accident:

> When Christopher Reeve fell from his horse he landed directly on his helmet, in a near perpendicular position, breaking two vertebrae in his neck. His spinal cord was not completely severed, but there was a large haemorrhage at the point of the injury. This damaged the nerve fibres that carry information from the brain to the muscles of the body.[25]

Reeve became paralyzed and then one by one, his organs shut down; unfortunately, he subsequently passed away. If pressure on Reeve's brainstem made everything worse, what do you think happens to people who have that pressure taken off their brainstems? That's right — they get better.

Imagine a truck drives over and parks on a garden hose; no water will pass through the rest of the hose and the garden will dry up. However, as soon as you drive the truck off the hose, water will again get where it needs to go and the garden will thrive. As simple as this analogy sounds, it is the reality. No benefit comes from pressure on the brainstem.

Once I grasped the reality of the power the brainstem holds, I no longer feared diseases. Truth be told, I didn't even know what I feared to begin with. I knew nothing about measles, mumps, rubella, diphtheria, pertussis, etc. All I knew was this dogmatic slogan: get your shots. For a long time, that was my mantra. Little did I know that when the brainstem is working properly, diseases stand little chance of harming the body.

From time to time, emergency medical procedures are necessary. However, those medical procedures and drugs are all too commonly overused. Let me use an analogy to illustrate how health works. Everyone likes a big, fat bank account. On a rainy day, when life takes an unexpected turn, you want reserves in that account to draw on. The same is true for your health. We all have a health bank account. When the nervous system is working at one hundred percent, it gives the immune system the best chance to work at optimal levels. A fully functioning immune system keeps you healthy and allows you to have reserves to draw on when you do come into contact with foreign invaders.

Several different events can cause the atlas to become misaligned. Chemical, physical, and emotional stresses can all pull the atlas out of alignment. Physical trauma is probably the biggest culprit and can even start at childbirth. The very act of being born can misalign the atlas. The act of pulling a baby out of the birth canal can be very traumatic. In other words, the toxic food we eat, the vaccines we get injected, the negative thoughts we constantly think, and the repetitive motions we make can all cause a misaligned atlas.

Let me make one thing clear here. Simply having the atlas in the proper position does not make you immune to diseases and/or infections. However, it does allow you to fight off those pathogens more effectively. When you catch a cold, if you do not stress the body out and you do things like decrease your sugar and dairy intake, the cold will last a lot shorter time and not be as severe. However, if you do the opposite, those stresses can pull the atlas out, and then you are behind in the game again.

I do not fear diseases. I fear not having my head on straight. And I do practice what I preach, as I'll show in these next examples.

When my son was four years old, he contracted pertussis (whooping cough). He had that loud, high-pitched wheeze followed by a deep, gravelly, raspy cough. It was cause for concern, and I needed to know for myself if what I believed was right. This really is where the rubber met the road for me. I knew that adjusting the atlas took care of headaches, neck and back pain, sciatica, and so much more, but this was whooping cough. I took him through the protocol to see if his atlas had come out of place. Unfortunately, it had. I gave him a specific upper cervical correction; the next day, his cough was gone. You can only imagine the relief I felt when my son woke up the next morning feeling well and ready to go to school.

My youngest daughter contracted measles. At first, we were not sure what the rash on her body was. The day after we noticed the rash, we took her to a naturopath, who confirmed we were dealing with measles. I checked her regularly to see if she needed a specific upper cervical adjustment, but it wasn't until the third day of seeing the persistent rash on her body that I realized the stress on her body is what had pulled the atlas out of place; she did need to be adjusted again. Three days later, the rash was gone. Through the whole process, she never ran a fever, acted lethargic, or had a decreased appetite. The only thing she had was a mild rash on her body, which ran its course, healed, and went away.

The power that made the body heals the body. In these cases, because the atlas was in the correct position, the body healed up just fine without the need for Western medicine.

I did not adjust the whooping cough or the measles out of my kids. I simply gave the body what it needed: a properly functioning nervous system. Please make no mistake; there is so much more to health than just having your head on straight, but this is a very large factor that oftentimes gets overlooked. Even having a nervous system working at one hundred percent does not ensure good health. If you were to eat at McDonalds for breakfast, lunch, and dinner for a month, trust me, you will not feel healthy. Likewise, if you inject toxic substances, such as the ones found in vaccines, you would not feel well. Our goal should be to trust that nature's homeostatic design will allow us to thrive. Vaccines do nothing to support your body's own homeostasis. If anything, they disrupt your body's ability to return to its normal rest state, thus creating a cycle of dis-ease. That translates into your body not being able to be "at ease." (For further information on this topic, refer to *Dissolving Illusions: Disease, Vaccines, and the Forgotten History* by Dr. Suzanne Humphries.)

Homeostasis is the body's ability to self-regulate. For example, if you get scared, your blood pressure rises. But once you are no longer scared, your blood pressure goes back down to its normal range all on its own. This is supposed to happen with all systems of the body. However, aluminum (a common ingredient in vaccines) crosses the blood-brain barrier and interrupts communication from brain to body by way of the brainstem. This can cause a global disruption for the body to then try to self-regulate.

Of the kids I see in my office, the ones who need the least care from me are the unvaccinated ones. Symptoms are usually different in vaccinated kids compared to unvaccinated kids. Vaccinated kids more often present with gut disorders, earaches, and more sleepless nights. Unvaccinated kids present with more musculoskeletal problems, typically caused by other siblings being too rough with them. And when those little bodies are "at ease," so are the minds and bodies of Mom and Dad. My sick daughter affected every part of my life. In a way, though, my experience was a blessing in disguise. It led me to see the world in a completely different way and from this, I am able to help others in ways I never thought possible.

My challenge to you now is to actually research everything. In my particular situation with Kate, she was sick enough for me to listen to anything and everything. I was willing to do everything necessary to get her better, but I knew that what I heard from the medical doctors was not the answer I needed. Again, I am not saying that medical doctors are not necessary; what I am saying is that if you are not getting the care you need, keep looking. A diagnosis is simply a symptom or group of symptoms lumped together and given a name. Usually a diagnosis is simply what you told the doctor translated back to you in medical terminology; this can give the patient a false sense of what is going on. But that gets the patient no closer to actually getting better. So *do* things to actually get you better. Life is always better with your head on straight.

04

FLOURIDE, 5G, AND FREQUENCY

By K.J. Moore, RN, BSN

"Without the conscious awareness of the dangers of 5g and fluoride, our human frequency is doomed."

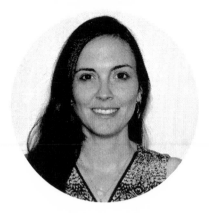

Kameren is a registered nurse (RN) with a bachelor's degree in nursing from the University of Southern Mississippi. For ten years, she has practiced in a variety of hospitals and units across the country as a professional travel nurse. Her healthcare expertise and broad understanding of the dynamics within the pharmaceutical and corporate world have given her an unexpected perspective on Western medicine. Throughout her career, Kameren has become more connected to health with a natural approach to medicine and mind, body, and soul healing.

Kameren's friends describe her as someone who is awake, driven, and intriguing. She thinks outside the norm and raises awareness of many pressing issues. In essence, she is an advocate for all people for health and wellness, for truth, and for Mother Earth. With so much corruption in the world today, Kameren is a beacon of light and truth for all those who dare to seek answers to some of the world's leading health and economic problems.

Kameren is a loving, compassionate person who enjoys spending time raising her children. She has six children, five of whom she birthed in the hospital and one of whom she birthed at home unassisted. Kameren has a passion for teaching and homeschooled her children for six years while working full-time as a travel nurse. She instills a love of reading in her children. Some of Kameren's favorite activities include exploring nature, hiking, and learning more about holistic healthcare. She loves making her own natural organic health and wellness products, which led to her opening an online shop where she sells items like organic elderberry syrup, CBD oil, and handmade crystal jewelry.

Kameren has always had a passion for writing and hopes that she can bring more understanding of real-world problems and solutions for a better future for our children.

www.carpediemnursing.org
ig: @TheWokeRN | fb: KJ Moore

My concern for the well-being and overall health of my six children drove my angst about radiation exposure and the inclusion of fluoride in our water and toothpaste, as well as some medicines. Why is fluoride being added to our water supply? Why are 5G electromagnetic frequency panels being put on water towers? My motherly instinct told me not to believe everything I heard about the health benefits of fluoride and the safety of 5G. The more digging I did, the more I realized that fluoride isn't as healthy for us as we once thought and that electromagnetic frequencies have never been proven safe either. In fact, there was insurmountable evidence that both fluoride and 5G are harmful and can cause damage on a cellular level.

Through extensive research, I started to notice some discrepancies. When I was a child, fluoride was not recommended by the experts until we were old enough to spit it out. Then when I started having babies, the grocery stores offered "Nursery Water," which is fluoridated water for babies. Why is it all of a sudden okay to give babies unlimited amounts of fluoride, while the instructions on the back of toothpaste advise calling Poison Control if toothpaste is swallowed? When I was a teen with braces, I was obsessed with brushing my teeth several times a day. Despite all my brushing, however, I developed a cavity that was bad enough that I had to either get a root canal or have the tooth pulled. My mom chose to have my tooth pulled, and I am glad she did because of the risks involved with root canals and their correlation with breast cancer.[26] Because of my obsessive brushing habits, my kids also had great dental hygiene. Yet as they got older, my seven-year-old son developed six cavities in his baby teeth! With all the fluoride in his water and toothpaste, why did my son have so many cavities?

After doing my own research, I was amazed to learn that our poor teeth are reflections of our poor health. My family and I had an unhealthy American diet at the time and lacked actual nutrients. Most of the food a typical American eats is either processed junk or made with ingredients that are unhealthy hybrids grown in soil that is nutritionally void of vitaminerals and humic and fulvic acids found in nature. My gut health was also poor from years of Western medicine. For many years, I was not aware of the use of detox methods to remove fluoride and other heavy metals from our bodies. I learned that instead of being beneficial, fluoride can actually be very harmful for us. I also learned that teeth can be remineralized to a certain extent, so I decided to make my own fluoride-free toothpaste, which I have been doing now for six years (check out the recipe at the end of this chapter!).

Not only do we have to protect our families from fluoride, we also have to be aware of the harmful frequencies and radiation in our food, air, and water. I will be discussing how a pesticide named fluoride found its way into our food, water, and medicine, how 5G electromagnetic frequency is harmful to us, and how to avoid all of the above.

WHAT IS FLUORIDE?

There are two distinctly different forms of fluoride. Fluorine, one of the most abundant gases in the earth, is a naturally occuring halide element found in the soil, water, and air. Then there is fluoride — an industrial byproduct of aluminum, a pesticide, and a known neuro-toxin. Since 1945, fluoride has been one of the chemical substances most commonly added to municipal water supplies with the intention of protecting our teeth from decay. While dental professionals once believed that fluoride strengthens our teeth and prevents tooth decay, recent studies have shown that it may damage organs such as the gut, brain, thyroid, and even the heart.[27] With all the heavy metals and toxins we are currently exposed to on a daily basis, is it really a good idea to be drinking and brushing our teeth with this neurotoxin? Even the FDA requires fluoride toothpaste to have a poison control warning label in the case of accidental overdose. This alone made me suspicious enough to research further into the truth about fluoride.

"Water is life, and clean water means health." ~ Audrey Hepburn

The History and Corruption of Fluoride in America

In 1931, H.V. Churchill, Chief Chemist of The Aluminum Company of America (ALCOA), discovered that populations living near water supplies with fluoride had mottled, chocolate-brown teeth, also known as the "Colorado Brown Stain." Because these people also had fewer cavities than other populations that were not exposed to run-off from the aluminum industry, the brown teeth were attributed to the water's high fluoride content.[28] Soon after this discovery, misinformation began to spread about fluoride's anticavity protection.

The highest consumer of synthetic fluoride compounds in the United States is the aluminum industry, which uses the chemical as a catalyst to smelt aluminum. For many years, aluminum companies had been searching for ways to dispose of sodium fluoride after use. According to the United States Environmental Protection Agency, "[f]rom 1973 until 1981, operators dumped tons of cyanide and fluoride outside the smelter on the ground."[29] This left our land toxic and poisonous.

Fluoride compounds were also used as a fertilizer and rat poison for over fifty years.[30] In fact, from 1896 to 1945, fifteen patents were placed on fluoride compounds for the purpose of pest control.[31] Sodium fluoride, ferric fluoride, and silico-fluorides all act as a contact and a stomach poison for rats and insects. Eventually the use of fluoride compounds as a pest control method faded out, while all attempts to use them as a fertilizer failed because of plant injury. However, fluoride compounds can still creep into well water due to run-off from farmland. Since fertilizer with fluoride was used for fifty years, much of it remains in our soil and plants, even in the food we eat today.

After all my research, it appeared to me that the aluminum industry and government were adding fluoride to our water supply simply to get rid of it. Avoiding cavities is not a reasonable explanation for brown teeth. In *A User's Guide to Understanding, Fallacy, Fraud, and Failure*, Bob Maddison explains:

> At the end of World War II, the US Government sent a research worker named Charles Eliot Perkins to take charge of the vast Farben chemical plants in Germany. It was disclosed to Perkins by the German chemists a scheme to attempt control any mass population by adding sodium fluoride to the

drinking water supply. This tactic was learned by German and Russian war camps to make the prisoners stupid and docile.[32]

Today, more than ninety percent of communities with water fluoridation use hydrofluorosilicic acid, a byproduct of phosphate fertilizers that was once considered toxic waste.[33] Hydrofluorosilicic acid also contains arsenic, which means the drinking supply in these communities contains heavy metals that can leach lead from pipes.

CRIME TIES TO FLUORIDATION

In addition to our water supply, many popular pharmaceutical medications are also full of fluoride and fluoride compounds.[34] Fluoride remains one of the strongest antipsychotics on the market.

A 2005 research report by Jay Seavey discusses the relationship between crime and water fluoridation in America:

> In 1999 I observed that nine of ten randomly-selected school shootings in America had occurred in fluoridated communities, and that the shooter in the tenth had used Prozac, a fluorinated pharmaceutical. With less than 60% of the U.S. Population fluoridated, a non-random correlation between fluoride and violence was suspected.

The report also references other scientists who connected fluorides with violence, stating, "several studies have examined the effects of fluoride on mental development, brain function, and behavior ... Fluoride by itself and in conjunction with heavy metals, appears to alter brain function and predispose some humans to violence."[35]

EFFECTS OF FLUORIDE ON THE BODY

When ingested, fluoride passes through the blood-brain barrier, which protects the brain and nervous system from damage by foreign invaders. Fluoride can even pass through the placenta to an unborn baby. While about fifty percent of the fluoride ingested is excreted through the urinary tract, the other half accumulates in calcified areas of the body, such as bones.[36] In addition, our water supply, farmland, food, and medicine all contain traces of aluminum, which is known to build up in the brain, causing Alzheimer's disease.[37] Aluminum is more soluble in fluoridated water, which makes it easier for our bodies to absorb. Other areas of the body affected by fluoride include the pineal gland, thyroid, heart, and gut. Fluoride also damages the mitochondria and depletes the body of iodine, which is important for growth and development.

One study showed that out of one hundred and sixty people who drank fluoridated water, fifty-two percent developed gastroenteritis. Another study showed that when forty-seven people were accidentally given excess fluoride in the water supply, ninety percent of them experienced nausea, vomiting, diarrhea, abdominal pains, or numbness or tingling of the face or extremities. One person died.

5G TECHNOLOGY

5G is considered the wave of the wireless communication future. It gives you faster internet — and is strongly linked to cancer due to hazardous electromagnetic radiation.[38] Electromagnetic radiation has never been proven safe for us in any stage of 2G, 3G, and 4G. While cell phone companies deny any dangers and cell towers are tested to be running below the government level of efficiency, 5G towers have recently been removed in elementary schoolyards in California due to a cluster of brain cancer cases in students and teachers.[39] However, the technology will be active across the nation in the near future, rendering the removal of these towers useless. By 2020, over twenty thousand 5G satellites will be connected to small antennas every 250 feet or so to ensure connectivity.[40] No one can hide from the harmful energy or "move off the grid" when this technology is connected.

5G technology relies primarily on the bandwidth of the millimeter wave (MMW), which is primarily between thirty and three hundred gigahertz (GHz) and is known to penetrate one to two millimeters of human tissue. MMW has been linked to a number of potential health threats, including eye damage, stress-related heart issues, arrhythmias, pain, suppressed immunity, and increased antibiotic resistance in bacteria.[41]

THE HUMAN FREQUENCY

Nikola Tesla said, "If you want to find the secrets of the universe, think in terms of energy, frequency, and vibration."[42] Everything is energy, and everything has a vibration. The Schumann Resonance is the frequency of the electromagnetic field of the Earth, also known as the pulse of the earth, and is generated and excited by lightning discharges in the cavity formed by the Earth's surface and the ionosphere. In other words, Earth is a magnet, and humans have a magnetic charge. The Schumann Resonance was steady at 7.83 Hz, but in 2014, the frequency rose and is now accelerating at 15 to 25 Hz levels; in 2017, it reached frequencies of 36+ Hz.[43] According to recent studies, frequency recordings of 36+ Hz in the human brain are more associated with a distressed nervous system than a relaxed one,[44] meaning the Earth is showing signs of distress.

WAYS TO AVOID FLUORIDE, DETOX THE BODY, AND PROTECT YOUR FREQUENCY FROM 5G

One of the best ways to avoid fluoride is to invest in a reverse osmosis water system for your home. While most filters remove every particulate except fluoride, a reverse osmosis system removes all particulates from water, including fluoride. If a reverse osmosis system is not in your budget, a more affordable option is distillation. Distillation removes all chemicals from the water. You may have heard not to drink distilled water because it has no minerals. This would be good advice if water made up your only source of minerals.[45] However, most of our minerals come from the food we eat. Municipal water supplies themselves are mineral-deficient and are in fact loaded with neurotoxins.[46]

Community water supplies have also been found to be full of unfiltered pharmaceutical waste and heavy metals, and bottled water is no better. Popular bottled water brands tested by independent parties have been found to contain fluoride and other unwanted substances.

For help detoxing the body from fluoride and radiation, there are some affordable and easily accessible options. Shungite is a carbon-based stone found only in the Shunga region of Karelia, Russia. Infuse between one hundred and fifty and two hundred grams of shungite in a liter glass of water for twenty hours; this will purify ninety-five percent of fluoride and other hazardous elements.[47] Detoxification can help protect our pineal gland (known as "the seat of our soul" and made of calcite microcrystals) from calcification due to fluoride, which is believed to lead to pre-pubescent changes in adolescent children such as lowered melatonin levels and quicker introduction to puberty.[48] Holy basil, also known as tulsi, has been used in India to defluoridate water and make it safe for human consumption. One experiment found that soaking seventy-five mg of holy basil leaves for a contact period of twenty minutes in one hundred ml of water removed ninety-four percent of fluoride.[49]

Nascent iodine can naturally detoxify fluoride and other halogens to which we are constantly exposed, including chlorine and bromine, as well as radiation and heavy metals including lead, cadmium, mercury, and aluminum. Iodine supports the lymph system, liver, kidneys, brain, bones, and thyroid and is responsible for the health of glandular tissue including breast, prostate, ovary, and thyroid tissue.[50]

Finally, hemp absorbs radiation and is known as a toxic substance vacuum cleaner, which makes CBD oil an excellent supplement for detoxing from fluoride and radiation.[51]

Upon realizing that our bodies are made of crystals and our bones are made of apatite crystals, I came to the understanding that we should be focused on protecting our frequency on a cellular level. Shungite also exhibits a unique shielding effect for harmful electromagnetic radiation from origins like computers, microwave ovens, TV sets, mobile phones, and 5G. Shungite, crystals, and metals combined in pieces known as orgone, or energy stones, can help protect your frequency from unwanted electromagnetic radiation and frequencies. In addition, you should limit your exposure to electromagnetic frequencies by turning off your WiFi router at night and putting your cell phone in airplane mode.

Since becoming more aware of energy, frequency, and vibration, limiting my exposure to electromagnetic radiation, avoiding fluoride like the plague, using shungite, and making my own toothpaste, I have seen a dramatic improvement in my health. My mental and physical health, as well as my children's health, have never been better. I am more physically fit and am accomplishing more than ever. My children and I have not had a major illness for which we had to visit a medical doctor in over seven years, nor have we had a cavity. The chronic fatigue I have suffered from since childhood is gone. I am finally doing things I always wanted to do, like starting my own business and working outside of the hospital.

With my new perspective, I could not unsee the lies that were passed down from generation to generation. Life doesn't have to be full of illness. We need to minimize exposure to electromagnetic frequencies and heavy metal neurotoxins like fluoride. Our children deserve the best, brightest, and healthiest future of all.

MY PEARLY WHITE HOMEMADE FLOURIDE-FREE RECIPE

WHAT YOU NEED:

- 1/4 - 1/2 cup of food-grade diatomaceous earth
- 1/2 - 2/3 cup of organic coconut oil
- 10 drops of organic essential oil of choice (orange, lemon, cinnamon, peppermint, spearmint)
- Organic stevia or agave to taste, if sweetener is preferred

INSTRUCTIONS:

Mix ratios to preferred consistency; do not use a metal spoon or container, as the metal will leach into the mixture.

NATURAL REMEDIES FOR ILLNESS

By Elizabeth Goebel

"Mother nature has lovingly given us all we
need to sustain our health."

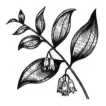

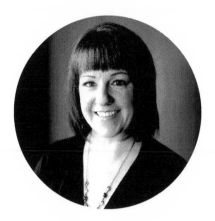

Elizabeth Goebel is an inspired, free-spirited soul on a quest for knowledge, truth, and love. She is a mother, blogger, activist, and aspiring holistic nutritionist and energy healer. She believes a positive internal dialog, faith, sense of community, exercise, meditation, holistic healing modalities, and whole, organic foods are the way to lifelong health and happiness.

Elizabeth once believed in vaccination and allopathic medicine (although her soul was always drawn to natural medicine). It was not until her son was vaccine injured at age four that she really dug into natural cures for disease and ways to stay healthy that did not involve pharmaceuticals with long lists of side effects. She knows that allopathic medicine has its place and believes that we need great doctors, but she also believes that we need to empower ourselves to learn about our bodies, how to keep them healthy, and how to heal them from illness or imbalance.

Now, after years of studying holistic modalities, Elizabeth is happy to report that she and her children are no longer on any pharmaceutical drugs and are living their best lives — happy, healthy, and free of disease! She penned this chapter with so much love in her heart, and she hopes that transfers to the reader. Her goal is to empower other parents to do their own research, find their own tribe of natural healers, and heal their own families, as she has done!

lizhealthyandwell.com
ig: @lizgoebel | fb: @elizabeth.goebel

"Nature itself is the best physician."

~ Hippocrates

This quote from Hippocrates reflects a belief and a way of life I have held for the last eighteen years. It only got stronger a few years ago when my son was vaccine injured and it was up to me to figure out how to heal him.

When my second son was born, he was perfect: healthy, perfect weight, loved to eat (all the time), bright-eyed, and just generally a great baby. My pregnancy went smoothly, and his birth went well. Slowly, his health began to change: breathing issues and trips to the hospital to get his lungs deep-suctioned because he often had bronchiolitis, constant runny nose, constant ear infections (so many that at six months old, he got tubes put in his ears), lots of crying (often high-pitched screams), and eczema. The breathing issues were so constant that at a very young age, our pediatrician hinted that our son had asthma. He was put on a nebulizer and prescribed albuterol; we used the nebulizer on a very regular basis throughout his early childhood. We had an asthma action plan by the time he was a year and a half. In his early years, our lives were spent watching and waiting for him to have trouble breathing, or for his skin to flare up, or for his ears to get infected (again). I was baffled as to why it was all happening. I was doing everything our pediatrician told me to do, and he was still so sick; our doctor did not seem concerned and said it was all normal, so we just went on and did the best we could to help our poor little baby handle it all.

A few years later, these issues were still ongoing. Then one day at daycare (where I worked as a preschool teacher), he began acting strangely. He was complaining of a tummy ache and headache and running around in circles, flapping his hands and crying: all of this shortly after receiving his flu shot and kindergarten shots. Finally he threw up; assuming he had a stomach bug, I took him home to let him rest. That evening, I left him cuddled up on the couch watching a movie while I made dinner. I asked him a question from the kitchen and he did not answer me. I spoke to him a second time: still no response. When I went back in the living room, he was staring blankly at the TV. He would not respond to me and could barely move; he was totally out of it. He just wasn't there. I immediately knew something was very, very wrong. We rushed him to the ER, and by the time we got there, he could not walk and was totally comatose. The doctors were baffled. He then started having what looked like some kind of seizure and lost all control of his bodily functions. The doctors intubated him. No one knew what was wrong or if he would make it. I was a mess, alternating between crying, praying, and vomiting.

My son was transferred by ambulance to a local children's hospital where all kinds of tests were performed. The next day, the doctors took him off of life support to see if he could breathe on his own. He did. He woke up, groggy but alive, and spoke to us.

The doctors said he had Coronavirus, which can sometimes cause seizures. They said it could have been a febrile seizure, although to my knowledge he had never run a fever. They did more tests, then more tests. Nothing. Everything was normal, according to their tests. A few days later, during yet another test, my son had another small seizure. It was nothing like the first one, which doctors called a "silent seizure." We went home three days later with a diagnosis of benign childhood epilepsy. The doctors put him on seizure medication and monitored him for the next few years. This medication caused a host of issues, such as weight gain and angry outbursts, and after a year of no seizures, we took him off of it.

I spent the next few years trying to figure out what happened to my child so I could make sure it *never* happened again. I knew some people in the anti-vax community, and one of them suggested my son could be suffering from a vaccine injury. I thought this person was absolutely nuts, but I was scared and willing to do my research. I scoured *PubMed* and Google Scholar. I read every book, watched every documentary, and talked to every person I could about the subject. I was shocked and horrified by what I found. Vaccines aren't safe or effective, and they absolutely could have caused everything that happened to my son, from ear infections to seizures.

I went over some of his medical records, and what do you know? Following almost every vaccination, he got sick! I was stunned. Next I found a group of doctors and chiropractors who would help him heal. My son's gut was a mess, and a blood test confirmed that he had sensitivities to nearly every food. I took him to an integrative pediatrician who understood vaccine injury and had been helping children heal from them for years. She clinically diagnosed my son as vaccine injured and said, "He is not a good candidate for vaccination." (And yes, other children in her practice are fully vaccinated.)

From there, we changed his diet, switched to an integrative family doctor, and started a program at our chiropractic office to address his vaccine injury. We've never looked back, and my son has never had another seizure or vaccine ever again. As of this moment, he has not needed his inhaler in almost two years, and he's not needed an antibiotic in about two years (except for a nasty case of strep throat). He rarely gets ill, and when he does, he almost always fights it off without medication. My commitment to heal my child, hundreds of hours of research on vaccination and natural remedies for disease, attending school for holistic nutrition, and spending time with a wonderful functional medicine doctor and group of chiropractors has led me here, to writing this chapter for this book.

Natural remedies are a time-tested way to heal your family using ingredients you can find in your kitchen, garden, and health food store. In my experience, you are what you eat, and a healthy diet full of fresh, organic plants and whole foods is the best way to prevent disease from occurring in the first place. Plant foods are high in antioxidants, which give the body the tools needed to fight off sickness on its own, while fermented foods, drinks, and probiotics, provide your body with much-needed good bacteria. Juices, freshly made from organic fruits and vegetables, are a great way to help your body heal.[52] Proper rest, plenty of exercise, and time outdoors are also important for overall health.

Regular chiropractic care is critical for immune function as well. According to one study, "[c]hiropractic adjustments can reduce stress placed on someone's immune system, freeing up energy to be used towards disease prevention and maintaining homeostasis. Chiropractic care aims to address the whole body, enhancing patients' ability to think, move and perform . . ."[53]

At the onset of any disease, one can start taking vitamin C (as sodium ascorbate, or liposomal) and vitamin D. Vitamin C stimulates the antibody response. You can take up to one thousand mg three times daily.[54] Researchers believe vitamin D offers protection by increasing antimicrobial peptides in your lungs. This is one reason why colds and flus are most common in the winter, when our exposure to sunlight (and therefore the body's natural vitamin D production) is at its lowest.[55]

The next step is to head to your local health food store and find a suitable immune system support. My favorite immune boosters are ones that use immune-recharging mushrooms, like turkey tail, sun mushrooms, maitake, lion's mane, and reishi, to name just a few. Research has shown that mushrooms, like the ones mentioned above, are antimicrobial, antiviral, antitumor, anti-allergic, immunomodulating, and anti-inflammatory.[56] You will have no problem finding supplements for immune health that include these mushrooms.

A variety of essential oils can also be used to boost immunity and ward off infections. My favorites are lavender, tea tree, and frankincense. These oils can be used in a diffuser, which creates a fine mist of antimicrobial molecules in the air. Diffusers can help keep others in the house from becoming ill while helping to clear the congested person's sinuses. These oils can also be applied to the affected persons feet, chest, wrists, and spine. Please consult an aromatherapist or other specialist before using essential oils on children.

Frankincense oil has anti-rheumatism, anti-inflammatory, antibacterial, antifungal, and anticancer activities, according to studies. I use frankincense diluted in coconut oil on the bottom of my family's feet and down their spines at the first sign of illness.[57 58 59]

Lavender oil has antioxidant, antimutagenic, anti-inflammatory, analgesic, and antimicrobial properties and can be used in conjunction with frankincense oil. A 2013 study found that lavender oil increased the activity of the body's most powerful antioxidants – glutathione, catalase, and SOD.[60]

Tea tree oil activates immune response and the accumulation of T cells. It is also antiseptic, antiviral, antimicrobial, bactericidal, and fungicidal and can be used in conjunction with the above oils.[61][62]

Below is a list of some of the diseases we vaccinate for (and therefore are taught to fear) and their natural remedies.

FLU

Echinacea root: Echinacea root stimulates immune-supporting white blood cells, T cells, macrophage, and interferon activity and shortens flu symptoms by a few days. It also has antibacterial and antibiotic properties. You can drink a tea with Echinacea root or opt for the pill form.[63][64][65]

Elderberry: Elderberry minimizes the duration of flu symptoms. According to a study published in *The Journal of International Medical Research* in 2004, ninety percent of people suffering from the flu who were given elderberry syrup felt better in three days. You can take a dose every few hours at onset of flu symptoms and gradually decrease the dose as you start to feel better. You can also take elderberry syrup daily during the winter months (cold and flu season) to ward off the flu.[66][67]

Ginger root: Ginger works to block the attachment of viruses to areas commonly affected by the flu first, like your lungs and airways. You can simply peel a small piece of fresh ginger and add it to warm water; I like to add a bit of honey to make it more palatable.[68][69]

Umcka: According to research, umckaloabo is effective as a treatment for acute respiratory infections, acute bronchitis, and coughs with mucus production.[70]

Eucalyptus oil: Eucalyptus oil is antibacterial, antibiotic, anti-inflammatory, antiseptic, and antiviral.[71][72][73] You can drink eucalyptus tea, take the herb in capsule form, or use as an essential oil on the chest (diluted in carrier oil).

MEASLES

Vitamin C: Vitamin C therapy helps with measles so you can load dose while symptoms persist.[74]

Vitamin A: Vitamin A therapy is the most common therapy for measles:

Several recent investigations have indicated that vitamin A treatment of children with measles in developing countries has been associated with reductions in morbidity and mortality. The World Health Organization (WHO) and the United Nations International Children's Emergency Fund (UNICEF) issued a joint statement recommending that vitamin A be administered to all children diagnosed with measles in communities where vitamin A deficiency (serum vitamin A <10 µg/dL) is a recognized problem and where mortality related to measles is ≥1%...Vitamin A is available in low-cost liquid formulations and is supplemented in infant formulas).[75]

Vitamin A helps regenerate T cells and supports the body's ability to create killer cells, increasing the immune response to antigens.[76] I opt for fresh or powdered carrot juice and cod liver oil to provide sources of vitamin A for my family.

Aloe vera: Aloe has antibacterial and cooling properties, making it perfect for all sorts of rashes and skin irritations. It can be mixed with a small amount of tea tree, lavender, and chamomile essential oils if desired for added comfort and healing.[77][78]

Chamomile: Chamomile is anti-inflammatory, antiseptic and emollient.[79] It can be added to bath as a dried herb and can also be used with aloe vera and applied to the skin.

Calendula: Calendula is anti-inflammatory and regenerative. It can be applied as a cream; alternatively, calendula tea bags can be used in a bath.[80]

MUMPS

Ginger: Ginger provides relief from pain and swelling associated with the mumps. It has analgesic, antispasmodic, and warming properties. You can use a paste made of powdered ginger and aloe (which is also soothing) and apply it to the face/neck two to three times a day to help with pain and swelling.[81][82]

Mullein: Mullein provides anti-inflammatory, antiviral, and demulcent (relieves irritation of the mucous membranes of mouth/throat by forming a protective film) properties. It can be taken as a tea or tincture to provide relief for the throat.[83]

Manuka honey: Manuka honey will soothe the throat and promote healing.[84] It can be added to mullein tea or warm nut milk.

Turmeric: Turmeric milk will help ease inflammation.[85] To make a "mump buster" drink, warm the milk of your choice, steep a tea bag of mullein, add Manuka honey and turmeric, and blend well.

CHICKEN POX

Don't scratch, just pat the itch. Colloidal oatmeal baths can be used to neutralize the discomfort, irritation, and itch of the chicken pox rash.[86] The same creams/oils/teas apply to chicken pox as to measles.

MENINGITIS

If you think your child may have meningitis, please contact your healthcare provider as this is quite serious. Do not try to treat your child at home on your own but you can give your child antiviral herbs, like elderberry and Echinacea, and antibacterial herbs, like goldenseal and barberry.[87]

TETANUS

Tetanus cannot live in a well-cleaned wound that has bled. The bacilli do not circulate in the blood; rather, they remain at the point of entry and release toxins. Clean the wound or puncture well with hydrogen peroxide, making sure no dirt or debris is left behind. Essential oils that kill bacteria, such as basil oil, lavender oil, sage oil, and tea tree oil, can be applied, as long as they are very diluted in either aloe vera or coconut oil (both of which have antibacterial properties on their own).[88 89 90]

WHOOPING COUGH

Vitamin C protocol: To treat whooping cough, you can use sodium ascorbate or liposomal sodium ascorbate. Use twenty to thirty grams for an adult and five to ten grams for a child, spread out throughout the day. This is a high dose, called a load dose, and is necessary to fight the infection. If you take too much, you will experience loose bowels (your body's way of getting rid of the extra vitamin C) and can slightly back off the dose the next day.

Eucalyptus: It is best not to give over-the-counter cough suppressants for whooping, as you want to expel the mucus from your body.[91,92] If your cough is severe and you need some relief, you can use eucalyptus to relieve the cough. This can be applied to the chest, diluted in carrier oil. Do not use eucalyptus on children.[93]

Marshmallow root: This is also a safe and effective cough remedy. According to Thompson and Camp (2017), "[marshmallow root] contains mucilage and antitussive properties that decrease irritation in the throat due to coughing, reduces inflammation of the lymph nodes, and speeds recovery from illness"…[94]

Honey and turmeric: Honey and turmeric can be taken for cough as well. Honey will help soothe the cough and loosen secretions, while turmeric will help with the inflammation associated with whooping cough. You can add one teaspoon of turmeric and one tablespoon of honey to eight ounces of warm water or nut milk a few times a day. You can also just swallow a teaspoon of honey every hour (this is not safe for infants under one year old) and take turmeric in pill form.[95]

A NOTE ABOUT FEVER

Parents have been conditioned to fear it, but fever is the body's innate mechanism to deal with disease.[96] Fever is an indication that your body is working hard to burn up pathogenic microbes, and eradicating the fever should not be your goal.[97] When my children are running fevers, we drink fresh, organic green juices mixed with coconut water (a great source of electrolytes) to keep us hydrated. A favorite in our house is pineapple coconut water.

It is important to determine whether your child's fever stems from a mild infection, like the common cold or the flu, or a more serious one, such as meningitis. If your child is listless, confused, short of breath, can't turn his or her head, complains of severe neck pain, or displays other disturbing behaviors with the fever, a call to your doctor is warranted.[98] Untreated fevers caused by viral or bacterial infections will not exceed one hundred and five degrees. Only in the case of heatstroke, poisoning, and other external causes will the fever reach or exceed one hundred and six degrees. If this happens contact Poison Control or get your child to the emergency room immediately.[99]

In my experience, it is important to trust a healthy body's innate ability to heal itself from disease. The suggestions in this chapter, which are based on research, are how I keep my family healthy, and I hope they help you keep yourself and your families healthy as well!

REGENERATIVE DETOXIFICATION WITH HEALING FOODS

By Melissa Weber

"The body has the ability to heal itself when given what it needs."

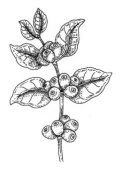

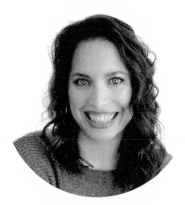

Melissa Weber is a registered nurse and successful entrepreneur who resides outside of St. Louis, Missouri. She is also a proud wife and homeschooling mom of three amazing children. Now that her children are almost grown and beginning lives of their own, her focus is on natural healing and helping others recover from illness and become whole again. Melissa began working with healing foods, detoxification, and regeneration of the body as a means to heal herself and her family. She has always had a heart for helping others and is currently in the process of becoming a certified detoxification specialist. Melissa works with ASEA, using redox signaling molecules with her clients and changing lives every day.

e: mlweber@myasealive.com

You've probably heard the famous saying by Hippocrates: "Let food be thy medicine and medicine be thy food."[100] But you may have never given it an ounce of thought. Well, now is the time to wipe the slate clean of any preconceived notions about what foods are healing and what foods are not. Throughout my journey to find the path to healing, I was struck with the realization of how powerful whole living foods are; food truly is medicine. Let me give you a little history of the road my family and I traveled to get to a place of complete desperation and how we began climbing out of the valley. I want to give hope to any of you who are merely treading water from all the damage being done by vaccinations and the food industry. Having a mustard seed of hope is everything, and having information makes us powerful in the healing realm.

I was a vaccine-injured nurse with vaccine-injured children. I followed the rules, not even questioning vaccines or considering the possibility that they could steal, kill, and destroy. As a practitioner of conventional medicine (which most definitely has its time and place), I had no doubt that I was doing the best I could for my family. My health began going downhill after nursing school, but it was subtle things such as anxiety, depression, fatigue, and a hundred odd symptoms no one could piece together. At the time, I never correlated it with vaccines. I suffered for about twenty years, living through hell on Earth before I almost lost my life. No medical professional could get to the bottom of my health issues, but I knew that the problems were not in my head, as some inferred. A few of the diagnoses/symptoms I gathered through the years included Lyme disease, co-infections (Coxsackie and Epstein-barr), heavy metals, mold toxicity, breast implant illness, neurological symptoms (tremors, buzzing, internal shaking), memory loss, loss of feeling in extremities, gastrointestinal distress, and chronic fatigue. I had lost my ability to walk and was completely bedridden; my life as I knew it was falling to pieces. Although these symptoms/diseases had names, I never wanted to identify with them.

Only now am I able to see how my illness became the greatest gift I could've ever received.

My awakening to the devastation of vaccinations didn't truly come until my husband and I found ourselves on the floor, performing CPR on our thirteen-year-old daughter. Every healthcare professional denied the DTAP vaccination could have caused a grand mal seizure and a diagnosis of absence seizures, but this momma heart knew better. This was just the beginning of many health issues for my daughter. It was devastating to realize I had unknowingly allowed this to happen to myself and my children. I wallowed in this devastation for many years and felt so defeated. I had no idea how to take back my power and start healing my family. It took almost losing my own life for me to start seeking real truth.

I thought I was doing everything right . . . I fed my family healthy, organic food as much as possible. Our plates were filled with a cooked vegetable, animal protein (grass-fed and antibiotic-free), and a fresh fruit. Still, my family was not healing. *How had we gotten to this place?* Google research had me in a never-ending death spiral most days and nights. We tried every supplement under the sun, and my lazy Susans looked like a natural pharmacy. But the disappointment remained so strong; no matter what supplement we took, we were no closer to the finish line. One day as I was spinning my lazy Susan in the kitchen, I remember thinking, "I should open my own supplement business." I'm sure anyone suffering and trying desperately to heal could say the same. This cycle went on for years.

In all my seeking of help from medical professionals and conducting my own research, no emphasis was placed on how powerful and crucial it was to consume whole, healing foods. The focus was solely on pushing isolated nutrients out of a bottle. I look back now and think, "Man, how did I not see it?" I was swimming in a sea of un-truths and barely staying afloat trying to heal my children and myself. But when you know better, you do better, and we have to give ourselves grace.

My healing began when I discovered redox signaling molecules[101] and started consuming them daily. At the time, I was deathly ill and praying for a miracle. I knew that my body needed help desperately and wasn't functioning at all at a cellular level due to all the toxicity I had incurred over the years. As my body took in the redox signaling molecules, I slowly became able to consume the healing foods I had once been unable to ingest and to utilize the nutrients my body so desperately needed.

Redox signaling molecules are native to the body and needed to help our cells communicate, repair, and regenerate; these molecules increase native glutathione (GSH) (the body's own master antioxidant/detoxifier) by over five hundred percent. Glutathione (GSH) is critical in the healing process and plays a multitude of roles, from increasing the immune system and supporting detoxification at the cellular level to joining with heavy metals to neutralize and remove them from the body to stimulate cellular growth, division, and repair and nutrient metabolism. [102][103]

Before redox, my body had pretty much shut down in the gut department. I could no longer consume any food except rice noodles, at best. Years before I became deathly ill, I lost the ability to eat most fruits. Touching citrus to my mouth left me bedridden for a month. I had no idea why my body was behaving like this or that I was severely toxic and acidic. Redox was a complete game changer. My severe brain fog began lifting; I was starting to put thoughts together when previously, there were days I didn't even know my own name. I added in new foods as my body would allow. Five months in, I was making small trips to the kitchen and back to bed. Once I was a year in, I could add some supportive herbs as well. My body was finally in deep healing mode and although I had some very trying days, these seemingly small accomplishments were monumental.

This is how I came to realize the power of living foods. I began a protocol that entailed drinking a pitcher of green smoothies a day, and let's just say that it was extremely eye-opening. I was not prepared for the healing crisis that followed. It humbled me. Truly, I had no idea how powerful raw foods are. This nutritional fact was hidden from me for twenty years; let's be honest, it is not common knowledge, to say the least.

Of course, not everyone will be able to jump straight into eating all raw fruits and vegetables. I had such severe gut issues that I had to start with only eating cooked vegetables and slowly work my way up to the raw foods. Detox and healing crises are real, and you must realize that the longer you have been ill or injured, the more unpleasant the symptoms that may occur while the toxicity is being purged from the body. This is a process, not an overnight fix.

Healing foods provide crucial supplies the body needs to put all the puzzle pieces back together again. The body is a self-healing vessel *if* it is given the right tools to repair itself. Our bodies desperately want to heal, but that healing is like peeling back the layers of an onion one at a time. The body can only detox and regenerate if it is supplied with the correct alkaline-forming foods that provide the proper vitamins, minerals, and hydration.[104] In the United States, however, the healing magnitude of food is practically a foreign concept. As a society, we are not told that when our bodies get the proper nutrition, they then have the ability to naturally heal and align themselves from the inside out. We aren't conditioned to treat illness with diet change. At the sight of the slightest illness, pharmaceutical medication is typically the recommended treatment route. But treating only the symptoms of illness will never eliminate the cause, and it's time to start spreading this message. Our bodies need foods in their whole form, not as isolated supplements.

Our bodies were divinely made and are miraculous machines, but regeneration cannot take place if they are continually being bombarded with toxic chemicals/vaccinations. Furthermore, the body cannot rise above this damage without first cleansing so it can begin rebuilding on a new foundation. Robert Morse emphasizes, "don't be fooled. Foods either feed, clean and rebuild you or they destroy you."[105]

The vitality of the human body is not solely based upon food consumption; it also depends on how much the body is obstructed by toxins and mucous.[106] Our body's main eliminatory organs are the gastrointestinal tract, kidneys, lymphatic system, skin, and lungs. In order for the healing process to occur, these channels of elimination have to be functioning properly.

One of the most vital systems is the lymphatic system, otherwise known as the body's sewer system because it is responsible for removing cellular waste. It is so important because "all diseases begin when this system becomes overburdened and fails."[107] The lymphatic system has to function properly to clean and protect our bodies. Environmental factors such as acids, mucus-forming foods, and vaccines can damage these organs and compromise the body's ability to detoxify and repair.

Another eliminatory channel that can be injured by vaccines is the gut; you can see where we begin going down this slippery slope while consuming all of the wrong foods our bodies need to heal. Start by eliminating mucus-forming foods, including all animal products, milk and dairy products, refined sugars, grains, beans, nuts, seeds, and cooked tomatoes, to name a few. These acidic foods should be reduced from the diet because they burn, inflame, and destroy our cells and cause obstructions, ultimately stopping the detoxification of heavy metals, pesticides, environmental toxins, and glyphosate altogether. This can wreak havoc on our bodies. The elimination of foods is just as important as the incorporation of healing foods to begin the removal of these obstructions.

Let's get into the process of alkalizing the body and discuss why food consumption is vital to detoxification and regeneration. Alkalizing foods consist of water-rich, nutrient-dense fresh fruits and vegetables that are unprocessed and uncooked. Feeding your body these healing foods allows it to start doing what it was meant to do, what it has been trying desperately to do. As you feed your body these vital electrolytes, they start alkalizing, hydrating, and energizing the body, which then enables the detoxification process. Alkalization equals anti-inflammation. Eat your hydration! Think fruits, berries, and melons. Some alkalizing fruits to focus on consuming include grapes, berries, melons, apples, cherries, mangoes, citrus fruits, papayas, and oranges. Some alkalizing vegetables to focus on include greens, spinach, seeded vegetables, cucumbers, bell peppers, beets, carrots, celery, romaine lettuce, peas, sprouts (alfalfa, green-leaf, and radish), squash, sweet potatoes, tomatoes, and white potato. Remember, depending on the severity of your illness, eating mostly raw fruits and some raw veggies is the best option. This is the most important part of healing, and what most healthcare professionals are completely missing — *the food!*

I also want to reiterate that healing cannot happen overnight. These obstructions may have taken years to accumulate, so removing them can take time, even years depending on the severity of damage. Focus on one day at a time as you feed your body back to life! You are essentially recharging your battery by consuming energetically live foods.

The detox pyramid is a must-know during this process. The higher up the pyramid you go, the deeper the detoxification. Cooked vegetables and leafy greens are at the bottom, then a combination of raw fruits and vegetables, green smoothies or green juices, one hundred percent fruit, fruit smoothies, fruit juice, mono fruit (a meal consisting of one fruit), and finally mono fruit juicing/water fasting and dry fasting at the top. This is a wonderful tool to use as you are healing and as you purge toxins. Don't be discouraged if you have to start at the bottom due to your health issues. I was so severe that I, too, had to start at the very bottom of the pyramid and work my way up.

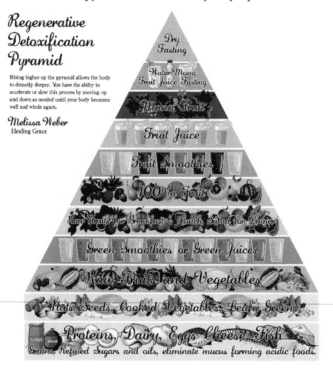

Regenerative Detoxification Pyramid

Rising higher up the pyramid allows the body to detoxify deeper. You have the ability to accelerate or slow this process by moving up and down as needed until your body becomes well and whole again.

Melissa Weber
Healing Grace

Dry Fasting

Water/Mono Fruit Juice Fasting

Mono Fruit

Fruit Juice

Fruit Smoothies

100% Fruit

Raw Fruits for Breakfast & Lunch Salad for Dinner

Green Smoothies or Green Juices

Raw Fruits and Vegetables

Nuts, Seeds, Cooked Vegetables, Leafy Greens

Proteins, Dairy, Eggs Cheese, Fish

Grains, Refined Sugars and oils, eliminate mucus forming acidic foods.

Fruits are amazing, beautiful, powerful healing foods when you are able to rise and move to higher levels on the pyramid. The sugars from life-giving fruits are the fuel that our bodies need to live in vibrant health and have naturally occuring energy. Fruits have the highest electrical energy of all foods on this planet. We've been told a heap of lies about these glorious foods, always shaming them for their wondrous fruit sugars. Trust me, I believed those lies like everyone else. But everything is energy, and our bodies need to be recharged by foods with high electrical energy. If we consume low-energy foods, it's comparable to a battery that cannot be recharged. Let me give you a few examples of the energy of healthy foods opposed to toxic foods. Cooked meats have zero angstroms of energy; cheese has eighteen hundred; cooked vegetables have between four and six thousand; fresh raw vegetables have eight to nine thousand; and fresh raw fruits have eight to ten thousand. You can see why consuming fresh, raw fruits and veggies recharges our bodies.

Contrary to popular belief, our bodies do not come from a place of lack. It is important to realize that we can't rely on vitamin and mineral supplements to regenerate the body at the cellular level. We must use powerful, life-giving foods because our bodies know exactly what to do with them. The simpler the foods we ingest, the better. The fewer foods you combine, the easier they will be for the body to digest. Our bodies expend a lot of energy during the digestive process, and if they are constantly trying to digest heavy, acid-forming meals, they won't be able to focus their energy solely on repairing and removing obstructions. Ultimately, we need to be able to digest, absorb, utilize, and eliminate properly — and that all starts with consuming raw, living foods.

Whole, living foods changed my family's life. They gave me back a life that I never in a million years thought was possible. My journey from sick and bedridden to alive and living was years in the making, but it was an eye-opening one that I vowed I would share if given the chance. Truth will always be persecuted and hidden; for that reason, I have made it my life's purpose to shine a light on this message. I pray it can be an immense blessing for your family and that you find peace in knowing others have gone before you. My prayer is that your family will no longer have to suffer and that this truth will bring you freedom, health, and wholeness.

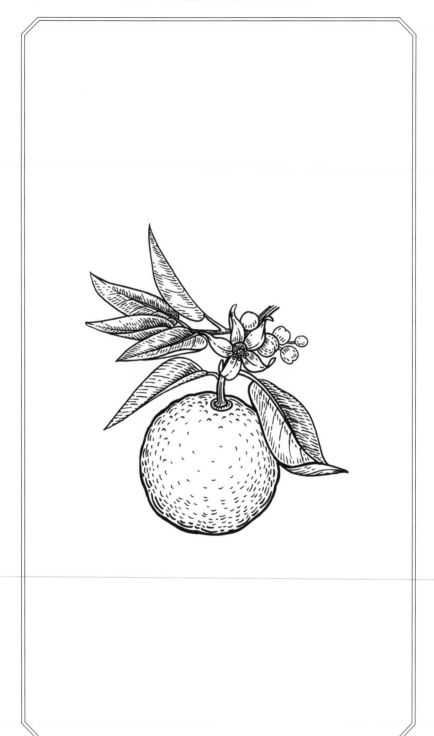

SIMPLE GREEN SMOOTHIE

INSTRUCTIONS:

- Pack blender tightly, three-quarters of the way full, with the greens of your choice (spinach, kale, etc.).
- Add fruit of choice for the last quarter of the blender to taste (fruits, berries, bananas, etc.).
- Add water, blend, and serve.

ORANGE BERRY SMOOTHIE

WHAT YOU NEED:

- Strawberries, blueberries, cherries
- Fresh pressed orange juice (press your own or buy cold pressed, non-pasteurized)
- Add equal amounts of fruits and enough orange juice for it to blend smoothly.
- Blend and serve.

SAFEGUARDING YOUR PREGNANCY AND BIRTH

By Suzzie Vehrs, B.S.

"The overmedicalization of pregnancy is creating sick mothers and sick babies."

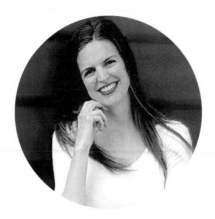

Suzzie is a mother, economist, and birth advocate. While at Brigham Young University, Suzzie had the chance to study the economics of public health. In this class, she learned how economists used statistics to prove that pollution was causing death in crowded cities. This led to a change in laws, cleaner cities, and companies being held accountable for the damage they were causing. It was here that she fell in love with the way numbers can tell a story and change the world. At the time, she thought battles like these had all been won. Five years later, Suzzie was a mom trying to help her child with a sensory processing disorder. As she met other moms on similar journeys, she heard the experience over and over: damage was happening because of vaccines. She pulled open her first vaccine book to do her own research, sure nothing could change her mind about vaccinating. However, after determining that everything she thought she knew about vaccines was propaganda, she knew she had to be a part of bringing this story to the world, to help the children suffering from the damage caused by our toxic choices. You can catch Suzzie playing at the park with her two girls, sneaking a salted caramel gelato while her kids are sleeping, and writing until 2am.

shebirthsbravely.com
ig: @shebirthsbravely | p: @shebirthsbravely

We like to think that we have the best healthcare in the world in the United States. *We certainly spend a considerable amount of money on it* ... so shouldn't we be among the healthiest people in the world? The truth is that despite our efforts to protect ourselves with more and more pharmaceuticals, we continue to get sicker and sicker. Our maternal and fetal health is among the worst of any developed nation.[108] The United States is the only developed nation in which the maternal death rate is rising. Thirty countries have better birth outcomes than the U.S. If there is ever a time to educate and advocate for yourself, it is during pregnancy.

One of the main reasons for the declining maternal and fetal health in the U.S. is the country's over-medicalization of birth. In our system, we use man-made pharmaceuticals and timelines instead of deeply studying, understanding, and working with the powerful forces of nature that are at play during birth. Some doctors entering the specialty of maternal-fetal medicine have been able to complete training without ever spending time in a labor-delivery unit.[109] To say that a lack of knowledge exists about how to facilitate birth is an understatement. That's not even to mention the conflicts that arise when you introduce the business-like hospital setting, which values predictability and timelines — neither of which are strengths of a natural birth.

Holding doctors as authorities on health when they may be totally uneducated about how to *create* health presents an enormous problem. One study found that less than twenty percent of medical schools require the suggested minimum hours of the study of nutrition.[110]

Although medical intervention can be life-saving in *some* situations, health will never be found in a shot. Pharmaceuticals that carry the risk of permanent damage and death should be used only after all other possibilities have been explored. Currently these interventions take precedence over lower risk alternatives that have proven to be effective at keeping people healthy, such as adequate nutrition, stress management, and proper hygiene.

Our children are being harmed and even dying because we have decided to look for health in a shot instead of studying life and living in harmony with nature. In the United States, babies receive twenty-six vaccine doses in their first year of life. This is the most vaccines given in any country. However, thirty-three countries have lower infant mortality rates than the United States.[111] This means that other countries are using fewer vaccines and have healthier children. Next time your doctor tells you vaccines save lives, ask them to prove it to you.

The United States has never conducted a safety study of the vaccine schedule as a whole. However, the VAERS database records vaccine injuries and shows that the more vaccines given to infants, the more infant hospitalizations and deaths are reported.[112] Our insistence on relying on vaccines for health is literally capable of killing our children. And it starts in pregnancy.

You and your child matter. As mothers, we demand better than this! Our doctors are experts at managing diseases through the use of pharmaceuticals. If you want true health and freedom from the side effects of pharmaceuticals, you must seek it out independently.

Let's look at the vaccines offered in pregnancy and the first hours of a newborn's life.

TDAP VACCINE

The American College of Obstetricians and Gynecologists currently suggests TDaP for all pregnant women.[113] Yet if you look at the package insert, you will see this statement: "It is also not known whether INFANRIX can cause fetal harm when administered to a pregnant woman or can affect reproduction capacity."[114] This means that we have no idea how this vaccine might affect a growing fetus.

There are *no* placebo-controlled, double-blind studies that show us the TDaP vaccine is safe to use in a pregnant population. In fact, we know that this vaccine carries risk for all people. The following adverse reactions, as found on the vaccine insert, have been found in a general population: bronchitis, cellulitis, respiratory tract infection, anaphylactic reaction, hypersensitivity, encephalopathy (swelling of the brain), headache, hypotonia (a child with hypotonia often takes longer to reach motor developmental milestones, such as sitting up, crawling, walking, talking, and feeding themselves), and Sudden Infant Death Syndrome (SIDS) (this one, to me, is especially scary!), among others.

Infant death and serious respiratory problems are known results of the TDaP vaccine; however, in the safety studies looking at birth outcomes for mothers administered this vaccine, babies who have died during birth are routinely excluded, as are those who spend time in the NICU.[115] Please reference this study published by the American Academy of Pediatrics as an example of a study that excludes the very population that could have been harmed by vaccines. This study excluded the non-vaccinated (who would be a perfect control), multiples, premature infants, and infants who died during delivery, among others (all of whom had mothers who were vaccinated). How is it that we allow a safety study to exclude the very population that was likely injured by the vaccine?

Most women are told the TDaP vaccine is especially important because of the whooping cough element. Yet reported side effects of the vaccine itself include bronchitis, coughs, and respiratory tract infections, all of which can be as severe and even life-threatening as whooping cough.

Not to mention that the current version of the vaccine, which replaced the dangerous DTwP vaccine, has been shown to be ineffective at preventing whooping cough. One study concluded that "all children who were primed by DTaP vaccines will be more susceptible to pertussis throughout their lifetimes, and there is no easy way to decrease this increased susceptibility."[116] The TDaP vaccine is not making our children healthier but rather paving the road for their sickness.

One more important thing to note: TDaP does not prevent *transmission* of whooping cough.[117] Many people believe getting vaccinated will protect the unvaccinated. In the case of TDaP, you can become an asymptomatic carrier of whooping cough even if you are vaccinated. Cocooning a baby by having everyone around him or her get vaccinated has not been shown to reduce cases of whooping cough.

FLU VACCINE

The insert accompanying the flu vaccine states, "There are, however, no adequate and well-controlled studies in pregnant women. Because animal reproduction studies are not always predictive of human response, Fluzone Quadrivalent should be given to a pregnant woman only if clearly needed."[118] Yet this vaccine is universally recommended across the board to nearly all pregnant mothers.

In a Cochrane review of fifty studies on the flu vaccine, it was determined that flu vaccination had no effect on hospital admissions, rates of complications like pneumonia, or transmission.[119]

The flu vaccine has not been proven to prevent severe illness or the spread of illness to the immunocompromised.

It is a shot loaded with risks. Mothers who receive certain strains of the flu vaccine during pregnancy are seven times more likely to miscarry if they have received it two years in a row.[120] People who receive the flu vaccine are also more likely to experience non-flu respiratory infections than those who have not not been vaccinated. This means that even *if* the flu vaccine provided you with any protection from the flu, your risks for similar infections have increased.[121] One study showed that if you receive the flu vaccine two years in a row, it *increases* your chances of getting sick with the flu.[122]

Talk about a misleading drug! No one should be getting the flu shot. The science does not show that it is safe or effective, and this is especially true for pregnant mothers who need to be extra cautious about what they are exposed to.

Now let's talk about interventions that will be offered to your baby.

VITAMIN K

The vitamin K vaccine is not actually a vaccine but rather a high dose of a synthetic form of vitamin K. This is administered to prevent a rare but very serious bleeding problem called Vitamin K Bleeding Disorder (VKBD).

VKBD can happen in three stages. Early VKBD happens within the first twenty-four hours of an infant's life. Classical VKBD happens within the first week. Late VKBD can happen up to twelve weeks after birth. The first two forms are rarely life-threatening and occur most often when the mother has been ingesting prescribed medications that inhibit vitamin K absorption, such as barbiturates, blood thinners, antidepressants, and antibiotics. Early and classical VKBD can also occur after events such as circumcision, birth trauma (such as forceps delivery), or other medical interventions.

Late VKBD is rare but can be very severe, even life-threatening. It has a twenty percent mortality rate and a fifty percent intracranial hemorrhage rate, which can cause mild to severe brain damage. In fully breast-fed infants who did not receive vitamin K at birth, the incidence is between one in every fifteen to twenty thousand. Late VKBD is almost never seen in formula-fed babies.[123]

The vitamin K vaccine is nearly one hundred percent effective at preventing VKBD. So if the vaccine is effective at preventing this condition, *why* would some parents opt against it?

The vitamin K shot has a black box warning, meaning that severe reactions, including fatalities, have occurred after administration, both intravenously and intramuscularly.[124]

There is evidence that the vitamin K vaccine could be linked to the development of childhood leukemia. Out of ten case controlled studies on this theory, seven found no correlation, but three did. The 1992 study that first pointed out this connection found a five hundred percent increase in the risk of leukemia when vitamin K was administered.[125]

If you are uncomfortable with the vaccine, you do have the option to administer an oral version of vitamin K.

THREE THINGS TO THINK ABOUT WHEN LOOKING AT VITAMIN K

1. Make sure you are getting plenty of vitamin K naturally throughout your pregnancy, using bioavailable sources. Vitamin K is stored in fat and transferred to the baby through the

placenta. Foods that supply vitamin K include spinach, Swiss chard, cabbage, kale, cauliflower, turnip, Brussels sprouts, avocado, banana, and kiwi. Cooking does not remove significant amounts of vitamin K from these foods. Nettle tea is also high in vitamin K.

2. Wait to cut your baby's cord until it has finished pulsing. This allows baby to receive more vitamin K-rich blood and stem cells.

3. Avoid taking medications that could interfere with your ability or your baby's ability to absorb vitamin K.

For the birth of my second child, since I had no increased risk of VKBD, I felt comfortable refusing the vitamin K shot and focused on getting adequate intake of vitamin K through my diet and postpartum teas.

HEPATITIS B VACCINE

Hepatitis B is a disease of the liver that mainly affects adults. It is spread through blood and semen. Most of the time, people acquire this disease through dirty needles or sex with someone infected. However, it can also pass from a mother to her child. Luckily, you can easily be tested for hepatitis B while you are pregnant. Most acute hepatitis B infections do not persist, but if the infection lasts six months or longer, it could lead to chronic liver disease, liver cancer, and death.[126]

The hepatitis B vaccine was originally made for at-risk adults. However, the community in need was not willing to receive the vaccine. After this failure, the scheduling of the vaccine was moved to be given to every child at birth. When asked to comment on this move by the *New York Times*, Dr. Harold Margolis at the CDC stated that, "This approach to immunize children to prevent serious chronic adult disease has never been tried before."[127]

Guess what — it's not working. *The Lancet* has reported that protection from the hepatitis B vaccine lasts about fifteen years. This means that just when that little baby may start experimenting with sex and is more likely to be exposed to the risks of hepatitis B, he or she is no longer protected by the vaccine.[128]

The hepatitis B vaccine also carries great and proven risk, including brain damage. As author J.B. Handley states about the effects of this vaccine in animal studies, "We have clear, unequivocal, replicable scientific evidence that the first vaccine given to most American newborns causes brain damage." [129] This vaccine is also linked to chronic adult problems, such as multiple sclerosis, chronic fatigue syndrome, systemic lupus, and asthma, among others. It has also caused anaphylaxis and Sudden Infant Death Syndrome in the short term.[130]

The hepatitis B vaccine does not provide lifelong immunity. It causes brain damage. It carries the risk of death and should only be given in cases where there is a risk of the infant being exposed to hepatitis B.

WHO IS DOING THE SAFETY TESTING?

No one is testing to ensure that it is safe to recommend these vaccines to pregnant mothers and newborns. *Informed Choice Washington* reviewed thirteen studies cited by the CDC showing the safety of vaccination during pregnancy, and *none* examined long-term impacts on the immunological, developmental, or neurological health of the child. Only two of these studies addressed vaccinations and miscarriage and/or stillbirth. Of those two studies, one compared low-risk vaccinated pregnancies to high-risk unvaccinated pregnancies, while the other is a meta review stating in its description that it is highly biased.[131] No studies have been done that give us any assurance that these vaccines are safe for a developing fetus.

In February 2019, the Informed Consent Action Network won a lawsuit against the FDA for failing to perform the safety studies required of the agency in order to recommend a pharmaceutical to the pregnant population. When required to provide documentation of the safety studies it had performed, the FDA responded, "We have no records responsive to your requests." Robert F. Kennedy, Jr., a vaccine safety advocate and lawyer in this case, stated, "As a nation, we can no longer pretend our trusted agencies are protecting our children. It is time to hold federal agencies accountable."[132] There is no one watching to make sure these vaccines are safe. If you opt to use them, you are the safety test. Next time your doctor tells you your vaccines have been thoroughly safety tested, ask him to provide sources and research before you accept.

PIECING IT ALL TOGETHER

If you decide to pass on vaccines, what should you do instead? Living healthy requires you to know how you fit in with the dance of life that Mother Earth sustains. Focus on these three steps to wellness:

1. Learn how to honor your cycles of rest, work, and play. Let your body rest, spend time in the sunshine, meditate or pray regularly, laugh often, and spend time observing your body and getting to know your signals of health and sickness so that when you do get ill, you can catch it early, when it is easiest to treat.

2. Deeply nourish your body with healthy, organic foods, especially fruits and vegetables. Remove as much processed junk and sugars as you can.

3. If you do become ill, use your judgement and the judgement of a naturopath, herbalist, dietician, chiropractor, or acupuncturist to see if there is a less invasive approach to restoring your health. Recognize that there is a time and place for pharmaceuticals, but the same practitioner who can slice and dice you or inject you with a shot may not know about how to use vitamins, herbs, or energy to help you return to homeostasis. There is not a monopoly on knowledge of health but rather a ladder of individuals who can help you at different levels of need and urgency. Become familiar with each of the diseases that vaccines supposedly prevent and find the vitamin protocols associated with them.

In our overly medicalized world, we have learned to fear. We fear because we do not know these diseases. We fear because we don't have the skills and habits to create health. We fear because we have been led to believe that we are powerless against disease unless we have a mighty pharmaceutical to save us. That is a lie.

Begin your journey to a natural pregnancy one step at a time. Ask yourself, "What one step can I take today to live a little closer to how I want to be?" Then celebrate as you do it. Do this again and again and again, and the next thing you know, you will have learned many new skills. You will know your body inside and out, you will have a strong personal relationship with food, you will limit your need for drugs, and you will see how you fit in the natural world around you. You will feel proud of your accomplishments.

It does not take a giant leap or a great struggle to live naturally; rather, it will be a lifestyle that emanates from you because it feels so good. As Lao Tzu once said, *"A journey of a thousand lifetimes begins with one step."*[133] Welcome to the journey.

NAVIGATING MEDICAL FORMS AND ADVOCATING FOR MEDICAL FREEDOM

By Carrie Lee

"We share our stories of vaccine injury and natural alternatives in hopes of providing a useful roadmap for parents navigating toward the same destination — raising healthy children."

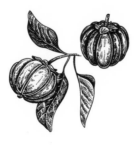

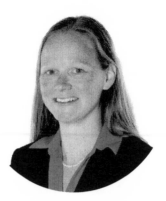

Carrie Lee is a married stay-at-home mom of three beautiful children, KC, KD, and CJ. Her family also includes their rescue dog, BB, and cat, Rainy. They're a small, close family that enjoys spending time together at theme parks and on cruises. Carrie was inspired to write her chapter in honor of her youngest son CJ, who was vaccine-injured. Her chapter focuses on exemptions, medical forms, patients' rights, and medical freedom. Since her son's vaccine injury, Carrie has learned vital health information and has become more conscious about the products she uses in her home. She has elected to take more natural approaches to health and beauty products and cleaning items and has ditched products with artificial fragrances to help reduce her family's toxin exposure. She started using essential oils and homeopathic remedies in place of over-the-counter medicines and includes other natural alternatives when her family is ill. Carrie has also become more aware of the food products she purchases; she tries to include more organic options, especially for dairy products, and avoids foods and drinks with artificial dyes. She feels it's never too late to change family lifestyles or life habits. She hopes parents find this chapter a helpful guide in their journey to natural health for themselves and their families.

ig: @naturallyinspiredmamasandpapas

fb: @carrieleenaturallyinspiredmamasandpapas

I was led to research vaccines and vaccine exemptions after the birth of our third child. CJ was perfect — born full term, alert, and healthy and began breastfeeding immediately. The day he was born, he received the vitamin K injection. Days later, he was given the hepatitis B vaccine at the pediatrician's office. Shortly after leaving the hospital and during his first week or so of life, CJ became lethargic and feedings were difficult. During his first few doctor appointments, I mentioned the difficulty I had waking him to nurse/eat, but his pediatrician wasn't overly concerned. After another two weeks or so, he was more alert and active so I didn't think any more of it.

CJ received all his two-month vaccines on time, and again we noticed he was unusually sleepy. Then, after his four-month vaccines, he would randomly start screaming a distinctively painful scream, and nothing helped calm him. Eleven days post-vaccines, I found him unresponsive, limp, and not breathing during the night. I picked him up, screamed his name, and jostled him to get him to open his eyes and take a breath. Immediately I thought, "Did my son nearly die of Sudden Infant Death Syndrome (SIDS)?"

The children's hospital admitted CJ for observation. After some testing, the results concluded that his heart was clear and he had no sign of infection — but that's all they checked. Although his pediatrician's office recommended checking him for seizures and apnea, the on-call doctor refused to do any neurological testing unless it happened again! She mentioned that they see these apparent life-threatening events (ALTE) often but they normally don't find the cause, and the event *usually* never happens again.

Hearing that it's almost normal for babies to stop breathing while sleeping with no known cause didn't sit well with me. I mentioned CJ had recently been vaccinated, but that was quickly dismissed by the hospital doctors as a possible cause. In my opinion, cognitive dissonance seems to be common when it comes to vaccine injuries. Our on-call pediatrician's attitude also changed instantly when I questioned vaccines as a possible culprit in CJ's sudden near-death; she did not return to the room after I asked questions, which left me feeling unsupported and uneducated.

This prompted me to conduct my own research. Like many parents, I was trusting; I fully vaccinated my two older children on schedule and blindly followed the advice of our doctor. I cannot recall discussions of risks or benefits, only instructions that my child would be receiving vaccines during the visit. I was handed a consent form to sign and a Vaccine Information Sheet (VIS) for each shot at the same time the nurse came in with the vaccines. I had no time to read these sheets or the opportunity to even ask questions before the vaccines were administered. Looking back, I would not consider this to be true informed consent.

Our oldest son has ADHD and learning disabilities, and our daughter suffered from a milk protein allergy and chronic constipation as a baby/toddler. I now constantly question whether vaccines contributed to these conditions.

Once I decided to stop vaccinating, I researched vaccine exemptions. I was shocked when I learned about certain ingredients in vaccines. I was unaware of the Vaccine Injury Protection Act of 1986, which James Turner, JD stated, " . . . was intended for parents of vaccine injured children to receive federal compensation on an expedited, no-fault, fair basis as an alternative to lawsuits. This act promised vaccine manufacturers that they were no longer liable for the vast majority of vaccine-induced injuries and deaths."[134] I was also unaware of the National Vaccine Injury Compensation Program (NVICP), which has paid out over four billion dollars in vaccine injury claims since 1988.[135] Severe and fatal adverse reactions are not rare, but the majority of these reactions are grossly underreported.[136] In my opinion, vaccine manufacturers have zero incentive to produce safe and quality vaccines; they're purely focused on quantity.

When I sat down to write this chapter, I was inspired to answer some of the most common questions I get from parents regarding my choice to no longer vaccinate my own family. Many parents either are not aware or are unsure where to begin when obtaining a vaccine exemption. First, I recommend finding a doctor who supports parental choice and medical freedom. Many pediatricians are stricter with patients who are not vaccinating, so keep an open mind toward family doctors and naturopaths. Second, review what form of exemptions are currently available through your State Department of Health. Current exemption options available as of spring 2019 include: Religious/Spiritual, Personal/Philosophical/Conscientious, and Medical.[137] Depending on the state and type of exemption parents are interested in, the steps vary and it can take time to complete the exemption process. Note that if you move to a different state, these exemptions will not carry over to the next state. Exceptions may include medical exemptions that are signed by a medical doctor or doctor of osteopathy; some states also require state approval[138]. Therefore, parents will need to begin the exemption process over again every time they move to a new state.

ARE VACCINES MANDATORY TO ATTEND SCHOOL?

Vaccines are currently *not* mandatory for children to attend a public school in the United States, in any state, at any school. As of early 2019, all fifty states allow for at least medical exemptions.[139] Follow the steps laid out in the previous section to obtain a state medical or non-medical exemption and submit it to your child's school. Be advised that due to provisions in many state laws, if a disease outbreak should occur at your child's school, your child may be required to stay home for an extended period of time, even with an exemption.[140] If a daycare or private school refuses an exemption, there are likely other schools you can try. Homeschooling is a great alternative if parents are having an issue with private or public schooling.

For college-bound students, contact each college/university of choice to request their Proof of Immunization Compliance to see their current requirements and possible exemption options; you should also research the states exemption laws[141]. Parents can also turn to helpful online groups for support and advice regarding their particular state. Most will happily assist parents through the exemption process, answering questions or even helping them locate a doctor who accepts unvaccinated patients.

MEDICAL FREEDOM

As of spring 2019, current vaccine exemptions in the United States, including medical exemptions, are being challenged at the state level in multiple states. These new proposed bills could even impact homeschooled children. I encourage citizens to stand up against vaccine mandates to help protect our medical freedom rights. We can help by being active with our state and federal vaccination programs, keeping up with potential bill changes, attending public hearings to voice our concerns about vaccine laws, and/or supporting rallying events. Search "health freedom + state" to find support groups on social media sites. You can also email, call, and meet with your local state representatives to share your viewpoints regularly. Parents should retain their right to decide what's best for their families. "Mandatory" means parents would no longer be able to opt out of any required vaccines, including the HPV or yearly flu shots. Parents would also lose control over what and how many vaccines are added to the mandatory schedule. When there is risk, we must always have a choice.

Vaccines were deemed unavoidably unsafe by the U.S. Supreme Court in February, 2011.[142] Yet the National Childhood Vaccine Injury Act of 1986[143] protects vaccine manufacturers from liability. The National Vaccine Injury Compensation program (NVICP) was created to compensate the children and families who suffered serious vaccine injuries and deaths.[144] However, Barbara Loe Fisher said:

I worked with Congress in the early 1980s on that (vaccine compensation) law and have watched it become turned into a cruel joke as two out of three vaccine injured children are denied federal compensation for their often catastrophic vaccine injuries because HHS (Department of Health and Human Services) and the Department of Justice officials fight every claim, viewing every award to a vaccine injured child as admission that vaccines can and do cause harm.[145]

This makes it nearly impossible for most families to even collect compensation through the NVICP vaccine injury court. Parents are faced with the nearly impossible task of pinpointing the proof that vaccines caused their child's severe injury or death, and most fail at proving their cases to the vaccine injury court.

Vaccines are not a one-size-fits-all philosophy because everyone processes/reacts to them differently, and some people may not be able to detox them properly. We can always vaccinate later on in life, but we can never take vaccinations back. Our children should never be force-vaccinated! Adverse reactions to vaccines can occur at any age and with any vaccine, including boosters. But even in the case of severe reactions, it's becoming increasingly difficult to find doctors who will write medical exemptions. Doctors may feel pressured to not write them or even fearful of repercussions if they approve too many. In my opinion, some doctors dismiss almost all reactions, including severe reactions, as normal. Perhaps these injuries are more common today, but they are certainly not normal, and a large majority of vaccine providers fail to report these vaccine-related health problems/reactions to VAERS (Vaccine Adverse Event Reporting System).[146] Even though the federal Vaccine Injury Act of 1986 requires vaccine providers/doctors to report recent hospitalizations, injuries, serious health problems, and deaths post-vaccines to VAERS, it is estimated that less than ten percent are ever reported. Parents can also file their own report with VAERS if their doctor fails to file one.

I fully support parental rights and vaccination choice, whatever those choices may be. We're all in this fight for medical freedom together, and we're fighting for the rights that parents may not even realize they need or want before it's too late. Forced/mandated vaccinations are unconstitutional because they violate our amendment rights, religious beliefs, and the Nuremberg Code Of Ethics.[147] In 2019, some cities in New York began to test these boundaries by trying to ban unvaccinated persons from public places or by fining Americans for not complying with a mandatory/forced vaccination. Some brave families are fighting back, filing lawsuits and hopefully setting a precedent that families will not be bullied/forced into compliance.

Online companies, such as search engines and social media sites, have also started to censor information pertaining to the negative effects of vaccines and/or the lack of proper safety studies. Some online donation companies are now refusing to allow fundraising efforts in support of anything anti-vaccine, while other companies are refusing the sale of anti-vaccine homemade goods. Some streaming services are even removing anti-vaccine videos and/or paid advertising from these videos.[148]

Things may get worse before they get better. But we must persevere, continue to speak up, ask questions, and advocate to protect our rights and our children, no matter how hard people try to silence us. Consider donating to organizations fighting to protect families' rights; you can also follow activists like Del BigTree, Robert F. Kennedy Jr., and Dr. Suzanne Humphries. The time is now to stand united for liberty and justice for all. Parents want true informed consent and the right to opt out of unwanted, unnecessary, and risky medical interventions. We must advocate for our state's rights, including the unethical dismissal of patients from pediatric practices for refusing to vaccinate per CDC guidelines and the use of vaccine-tracking databases that violate families' right to privacy. For a more in-depth discussion regarding the vaccination debate, I'd recommend the book *Vaccine Epidemic.*

VACCINATION REFUSAL FORMS

If parents have decided to refuse vaccinations or delay the schedule, they may be asked to sign a Vaccination Refusal Form. I encourage parents to familiarize themselves with this form beforehand.[149] These forms often imply that parents are potentially harming their child and endangering their community by refusing vaccines. The doctor/nurse or office staff may try to use pressure, fear, or intimidation to get parents to comply and sign before they leave the office. However, regardless of what the office staff implies, parents always have the legal right to opt out of signing these potentially incriminating forms.

The only drawback to not signing this form is that the doctor's office may tell parents to find a new doctor. The trend of dismissing patients for refusal to follow the CDC vaccine schedule is increasing, making it nearly impossible for some parents to find primary pediatric care. Most pediatric offices require refusal forms, which can differ from office to office. Most importantly, never feel rushed or forced to sign without the opportunity to carefully review and understand the form first. Instead, you can ask to take the form home, where it's easier to review without any distractions from a child or office staff. Sometimes when parents refuse to sign, the nurse can just notate "parent refusal on the form." Another option is to completely cross out any statements implying that parents are putting their child or others in harm's way by refusing vaccines; just make sure to initial each time a change is made on the form.[150] If the form is rejected due to the removal of incriminating statements that the parents disagree with, then parents could try writing above the signature line, "I do not agree with all of the above statements" and sign.[151] If the office still refuses to accept the form, keep the rejected form as proof they would not accept it with any corrections.[152]

Parents can sign the form if they're one hundred percent in agreement with everything the form implies or if they're comfortable with the changes they made to alter the form and the staff has no objections with these changes. But offices may require a new signature every time vaccines are declined. Look out for any changes in the wording before deciding to re-sign a refusal form.

Parents can also prepare by bringing along their own Vaccination Notice Form.[153] Another option is to bring along a copy of a Physician's Warranty of Vaccine Safety form to your doctor. If the doctor refuses to sign it, then the Vaccination Notice Form is a good compromise for both parties. Since vaccinating and not vaccinating both carry risks of potential harm, this form protects the parents and the doctor. However, if parents feel like their hands are tied and they are forced to sign the refusal form, they can sign it under duress; for this reason, I advise you to bring a witness with you, such as a family member or supportive friend.[154] Parents may be able to rescind their signature on a vaccination refusal form.[155]

Wellness/vaccination appointments and refusal forms can feel overwhelming, especially for new parents, but keep in mind that doctors work for us. We hire them and we can fire them. If you have any doubt at these appointments, don't react just yet. Go home, think about it, and research more. You can come back better prepared to discuss things at future visits.

Remember, a doctor should never force, scare, or belittle parents into vaccinating a child. If parents do experience this type of coercive behavior, they can file a complaint with their state medical board. Parents are also free to get up and leave at any time, especially if they are being bullied or threatened. I expect gentle guidance, respect, and informed consent from doctors even if we disagree. Parents should feel comfortable asking their doctor any questions without the doctor becoming defensive or annoyed. Parents can even prepare themselves by researching "Effective Persuasion Without Confrontation Techniques," which some pediatricians may use to pressure them to vaccinate.[156]

Parents never need to defend their decision when refusing vaccines. In fact, defensiveness could make it easier for the doctor/nurse to try to sway the parent's decision. Instead, you could respond with, "We have educated ourselves on the risks and benefits and have made an informed decision not to vaccinate." Wellness checks should be a positive experience, and parents should feel comfortable addressing any concerns they have with their doctor. They should not fear their doctor. Parents are also encouraged to forgo signing any type of electronic medical forms and to request a hard copy instead. I'd also recommend researching biogenics/biologics.[157 158]

The current CDC vaccine schedule has never been tested in a long-term, control-based study with true blind placebos, nor has it been tested for safety in combination.[159] Children today are the test study, and only years/decades down the road will we fully understand all the side effects and risks associated with this ever-increasing vaccine schedule. In fact, Robert F. Kennedy Jr. said, "The CDC is not an independent agency. It is a vaccine company." He also said, "50% of CDC's budget goes to selling and promoting vaccines. CDC owns 57 vaccine patents and collects money on them." Vaccine advertising has heavily increased, and it's nearly impossible to not see or hear daily ads promoting vaccines. How can we trust a company that profits from the sale of vaccines?

OPTIONS FOR VACCINATION REFUSAL FORMS:

- Refuse to sign.
- Ask the nurse to note that you declined.
- Take the form home to review and possibly return.
- Replace with a Vaccination Notice Form.
- Cross out all statements you disagree with, initial changes, and sign.
- Write above signature line, "I do not agree with all the above statements" and sign.
- Sign under duress.

PARENTS' INTERVIEW QUESTIONNAIRE FOR DOCTORS:

- What is the doctor's philosophy regarding vaccinations, breast-feeding, alternative medicine, co-sleeping, and the cry it out method?
- Do they accept unvaccinated patients or support delayed vaccinations?
- Do they require a signed vaccination refusal form to be seen?
- Do they allow other guardians to bring children to appointments and make medical decisions, even if these guardians do not support parents' wishes regarding things like vaccinations, without contacting parents for consent?
- Chiropractors, family, and naturopathic doctors are a great alternative if parents have trouble finding a pediatrician who is supportive.

NATURALLY INSPIRED MAMAS AND PAPAS

There are other ways to build a natural and healthy immune system besides injecting diseases/infections into our children. In my opinion, babies are not born deficient in what they need to survive, and most medical interventions after birth seem unnecessary today. We need to step back in time and reflect on our ancestors' tried-and-true natural remedies. Natural health is not often found in today's mainstream medicine; it's also much harder to trust today's store-bought products and foods and to decipher the loopholes companies use to make these products appear safer/healthier. Healthy starts at home. Let's take back our health and wellness by growing our own herbs and foods and making our own products so we know exactly what's going into our bodies.

Here's the bottom line: if vaccines were safe and effective, doctors and politicians wouldn't need to mandate/force them, grant blanket immunity to vaccine manufacturers, or feel threatened by parents who question them. Shouldn't today's generation of children be healthier, not sicker, with the advancements in modern medicine? Instead, Robert F. Kennedy, Jr. points out, "Today, 54% of American children have one or more chronic health problems like ADHD, asthma, seizures, deadly food allergies and developmental disabilities. Published peer-reviewed scientific literature links all these diseases to vaccines."[160]

I guess, why create cures when they can create lifelong customers?

It seems the pharmaceutical industry profits more if we're ill and dependent on prescription medications. It's a vicious cycle in which we suddenly need more and more prescriptions to relieve new symptoms caused by the previous medication, and so on. Healthy individuals are not profitable enough, and even natural treatments cut into these companies' profits.

Doctor's visits were originally used for emergencies only. Minor illnesses and injuries were treated naturally at home. My hope for our future is that we retain our medical freedom and religious/personal exemptions, that proper safety studies are finally performed by a true independent agency, that vaccine manufacturers can be held liable again, and that no more children or families have to endure severe vaccine injuries and/or death. Parents call the shots, and no child should ever be sacrificed for the so-called "greater good!"

#EducateBeforeYouVaccinate
#WeDid
#WeDoNotConsent

SEVEN MYTHS ABOUT INFLUENZA AND THE FLU VACCINE

By Jennifer Schmid, MSN, RN, CNL, PHN, ACN

"A well-meaning parent who refuses to let her vaccinated asthmatic child play with a healthy unvaccinated child is not only depriving her child of a friend but also basing her opinion on scientifically incorrect information."

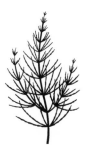

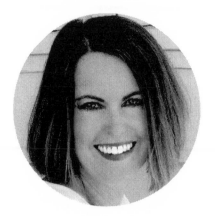

The founder of Oasis Wellness, Jennifer Schmid, MSN, RN, CNL, PHN, ACN, is a nurse and traditional naturopath on a mission to transform the way we heal our body, mind, and spirit. She bridges the worlds of conventional and alternative medicines, empowering people to take control of their health naturally and joyfully.

When Jennifer was in her twenties, doctors proclaimed that she would have to live with her chronic health issues because there was nothing they could do. She began studying and applying the principles of nature-based therapies, healed herself of an "incurable" condition, and has never looked back.

Jennifer creates a safe, supportive space for consumers and healthcare practitioners to learn about evidence-based alternative solutions and options that help people where they're at. Everyone should be able to heal in a way that makes them feel good without miserable (or deadly) negative side effects. With a customized and humanized approach to healing, Jennifer is shattering the old patriarchal pharmaceutical paradigm to make way for twenty-first century *health* care.

Jennifer is the proud mom of three amazing young adults and is currently based in California.

www.earthbasedmedicine.com

The flu season is coming! The flu season is coming!

Every August in the United States, we start seeing advertisements and hearing news reports about the impending "flu season." The fear-based messaging is always the same — death and destruction are going to rain down upon us from December 1 to March 31. The marketing tells us our only hope is to get our flu shot, also known as the influenza vaccine, as soon as possible; then we will be magically protected until the "flu season" ends.

We commonly hear these claims from the media:

- Thousands of people die every year from influenza.
- We have to get the influenza vaccine every year so that everyone is totally protected against getting the flu and giving it to others.
- We are helpless against influenza if we don't get vaccinated.
- The influenza vaccine is extremely safe.

The lack of evidence supporting the safety and effectiveness of the influenza vaccine makes it challenging for me to recommend the vaccine to anyone, but you need to make that decision for yourself and your family. It is a highly personal matter. I will share with you several common myths about influenza and the influenza vaccine to help you make your choice.

MYTH #1: INFLUENZA KILLS TENS OF THOUSANDS OF PEOPLE EVERY YEAR.

According to the CDC itself, "CDC does not know exactly how many people die from seasonal flu each year."[161] If that's the case, then why did *The New York Times* report that over 80,000 people died from influenza during the 2017-2018 season based on a press release of estimated deaths from the government's National Foundation for Infectious Disease, a national non-profit created to promote vaccinations?[162] [163]

Rather, the CDC estimates the number of people it thinks *might* have died from influenza-related complications:

> CDC uses two categories of underlying cause of death information listed on death certificates: pneumonia and influenza (P&I) causes and respiratory and circulatory (R&C) causes. CDC uses statistical models with records from these two categories to make estimates of influenza-associated mortality.[164]

There are two major problems with the CDC's methods of calculations:

1. Many patients with upper respiratory infections and pneumonia are not usually tested to see whether or not they have influenza. According to the CDC, "Most people with flu symptoms are not tested because the test results usually do not change how you are treated."[165]

2. Patients with chronic diseases such as congestive heart failure and diabetes often are lumped into influenza deaths during "flu season" because a respiratory infection like influenza could potentially exacerbate their disease. Similarly, say someone dies of aspiration pneumonia, meaning that a small particle of food got into their lungs, which then got infected and killed them. These patients still fall into the same category of deaths as those who died from influenza.[166]

So how do scientists, healthcare providers, and regular citizens know which patients died from influenza-related causes and which ones didn't?

MYTH #2: THE FLU VACCINE IS THE MOST EFFECTIVE WAY TO PREVENT INFLUENZA AND INFLUENZA-LIKE SYMPTOMS.

'EFFICACY' VS. 'EFFECTIVENESS'

Before we can bust this myth, we have to define "efficacy" and "effectiveness" because pharmaceutical companies and the CDC use these words to make us think their products work better than they actually do.

A vaccine's or drug's efficacy does not necessarily translate into how effective it is. Efficacy means how well a vaccine or drug works in the *ideal* setting — namely, a clinical trial — when scientists can control for all sorts of variables. Effectiveness, on the other hand, means how well a vaccine or drug works in the messy real world.

When reading scientific studies (especially those funded by a drug company), remember that a drug's effectiveness is *always* lower than its efficacy because there are always real-life variables that a trial cannot control.

In 2018, the CDC created its own definition of effectiveness for the flu vaccine: "The flu vaccine reduce(s) a person's overall risk of having to seek medical care at a doctor's office for flu illness."[167] This doesn't define the vaccine's effectiveness as actually preventing the illness it's supposed to prevent. Rather, effectiveness is defined here based on how "sick" a person feels. That way the experts can change their "mathematical models" to make the vaccine seem more effective than it really is.

Why did the CDC have to change the definition of the vaccine's effectiveness? Part of the reality is that scientists are not psychic. They have to predict which viruses might be the most prevalent (causing the most cases of influenza) and virulent (harmful) for the next flu season, and they have to do it rather quickly. The Food and Drug Administration (FDA) actually chooses which strains of viruses, such as H1N1 or H3N2, to put into vaccines based on "surveillance," "research," and "availability of vaccine viruses."[168]

Even though the vaccine propaganda says that the vaccine works to prevent flu, science has said otherwise. According to *Cochrane Database of Systematic Reviews (CDSR)**, which is the leading journal and

---

* Until very recently, the *Cochrane Database of Systematic Reviews* contained the most respected and impeccable analyses of research in healthcare. Through systematic reviews, they would review multiple scientific studies on a particular topic, such as the flu vaccine. However, in September 2018, one of their board members, Peter Goetzsche, was voted off of the governing board because he publicly questioned the accuracy of their review of the HPV vaccine.[191] Three other board members resigned in protest, and the validity of the CDSR reviews is now in question.[192 193 194]

database for systematic reviews, there is no evidence that vaccines help to prevent influenza or influenza-like illness in children under the age of two years old, regardless of whether the vaccines use a "live" or "killed" virus.[169] This same study also noted that in children of all ages, there was no "evidence of effect on secondary cases, lower respiratory tract disease, drug prescriptions, otitis media [ear infection] and its consequences and socioeconomic impact." This means that a well-meaning parent who refuses to let her vaccinated asthmatic child play with a healthy unvaccinated child is not only depriving her child of a friend but also basing her opinion on scientifically incorrect information.

The Cochrane review also called out researchers and pharmaceutical companies for deceiving both the public and the scientific community: "There is evidence of widespread manipulation of conclusions and spurious notoriety of the [industry-funded] studies." Translation? The "scientific" studies behind the flu vaccine cannot be considered valid or unbiased.

Now let's look at the injuries (also known as "adverse effects") caused by the influenza vaccination and the paucity of safety research.

MYTH #3: INFLUENZA VACCINES ARE THOROUGHLY TESTED FOR SAFETY FOR ALL AGE GROUPS BEFORE MASS DISTRIBUTION IN THE MARKETPLACE.

According to the CDC, "there has been extensive research supporting the safety of flu vaccines."[170] However, much of the research supporting vaccine safety is at least twenty years old and was funded by the pharmaceutical industry, which has a reputation for putting profits before public health.[171] This makes one question their definition of "safe."

VACCINE 'SAFETY'

Let's pause for a moment to talk about vaccine "safety." The United States' Federal Drug Administration (FDA) classifies vaccines as "biologics" rather than traditional pharmaceutical drugs. This makes sense because vaccines contain recombinant DNA (genetic material that has been artificially combined) and tissues from animals and humans. Once a vaccine product has been created, it is then cultured to grow in biological material such as egg, insect, or dog cells.

The initial safety testing process is supposed to be the same for biologics and chemical drugs, but there is one important difference. Once the manufacturing process for a vaccine has been approved and licensed, *that vaccine never has to undergo safety testing again.*[172]

Let's say that a pharmaceutical company named Big Pharma got a license to manufacture a flu vaccine in 1990. So long as Big Pharma uses the same manufacturing process (i.e., they continue to culture the vaccines in egg cells rather than changing to dog cells), they can make a new flu vaccine year after year without testing that vaccine for safety. In these yearly vaccines, Big Pharma can combine whatever viruses the CDC and WHO tell them to, plus whatever combination of preservatives they choose, but they don't have to test them annually for safety. Why not? Because *the product is already assumed to be safe.*[173]

This is why package inserts for the yearly influenza vaccines only discuss efficacy in their clinical trials, rather than including any information on safety. For some influenza vaccines, the original safety trials date back to the year 2000 and earlier. Additionally, *none of the individual biological ingredients or culturing mediums has ever been tested for short- or long-term safety.*[174]

To date, no flu vaccine has been recalled due to adverse events or for safety reasons despite growing evidence that such recalls may be warranted.

Most doctors, nurses, and pharmacy techs giving the flu shot know little about vaccine safety or adverse reactions. They rely on what they are told by the CDC. The reality is, the safety of the influenza vaccine is yet another unproven medical theory. Without large-scale, *independently* funded research comparing outcomes in those vaccinated against outcomes in those who are not, and without doctors willing to acknowledge and report adverse reactions to the Vaccine Adverse Event Reporting System (VAERS), we will never know the truth about influenza vaccine safety. We do know that acute adverse reactions, such as Guillain-Barré Syndrome, can appear up to six weeks after vaccination, but this information is not widely disseminated to healthcare practitioners and those who administer vaccines.[175]

CHILDREN UNDER TWO YEARS OF AGE

The 2012 Cochrane review shared that there has been only one study in children under two, using a vaccine proven to be worthless.[176] Worse, "extensive evidence of reporting bias of safety outcomes from trials of live attenuated influenza vaccines impeded meaningful analysis."[177]

Therefore, at this time, all the promises from the CDC and pediatricians that is safe to inoculate infants and toddlers under age two with influenza are not based on science.

CHILDREN AGED TWO TO SIXTEEN YEARS OLD

Influenza vaccination in children has been associated with permanent cataplexy and narcolepsy, as well as febrile seizures.[178] Cataplexy means that the child suddenly loses all voluntary muscle control, usually when triggered by emotions such as excitement or joy. This condition often partners with narcolepsy, which causes a disruption in the normal sleep-wake cycle and leads to excessive sleepiness during the daytime. Both cataplexy and narcolepsy are signs of severe neurological damage caused by the ingredients in the influenza vaccine, and they're permanent. The biological manufacturing process, bias, and lack of standardization in studies make it impossible to assess influenza vaccine safety in children before the vaccines are released for mass public use.

Likewise, the American Thoracic Society noted in 2009 that children who received the influenza vaccine were three times more likely to be hospitalized for the flu, and that the risk was even higher in children with asthma.[179] The authors of the study blamed the efficacy of the flu vaccine rather than the vaccine contents, but could something be happening to cause children's immune systems to react more severely to influenza *after* vaccination? Another study reported that children who receive the flu vaccine are 4.4 times more at risk of coming down with a non-influenza respiratory infection.[180] Why? Possibly because "annual vaccination against influenza virus hampers the development of virus specific CD8+ T cell immunity in children," meaning that the immune systems of children who were vaccinated against influenza had a more difficult time fighting other viruses.[181]

Most conventional researchers and people in the medical field refuse to acknowledge these issues. However, parents of children injured by the flu vaccine can tell you exactly what has happened to their child. It would behoove those of us in healthcare to listen to them.

ADULTS AGE EIGHTEEN TO SIXTY-FOUR

Just as with children, there are no clinical trials that look at the influenza vaccine in terms of safety for this age group. Instead, studies only look at efficacy, and *maybe* record some of the safety concerns. The CDC itself admits that most of our data regarding vaccine safety is reported to VAERS after a product has already been distributed for mass public use and that underreporting of adverse reactions is a serious concern.[182] We have plenty of reasons to be concerned about the safety of influenza vaccination in adults.

And article in the *International Journal of Obesity* states:

> Vaccinated obese adults are twice as likely to develop influenza and influenza-like illness compared to healthy weight adults. This finding challenges the current standard for correlates of protection, suggesting use of antibody titers to determine vaccine effectiveness in an obese population may provide misleading information.[183]

The CDC says that forty percent of American adults are obese, meaning that approximately forty percent of vaccinated American adults have been given a false sense of security when getting the flu vaccine. What is happening to the immune system of an obese person who gets the flu vaccine that would make them more susceptible to influenza, even when blood tests show that they should be immune to it?

We also know that the toxic ingredients in vaccines for diseases such as influenza, hepatitis B, and HPV can breach the blood-brain barrier and cause demyelination of nerve cells called neurons, resulting in cases of Guillain-Barré Syndrome (Acute Inflammatory Demyelinating Polyneuropathy, or AIDP), clinically isolated syndrome (CIS), acute disseminated encephalomyelitis (ADEM), and chronic disseminated encephalomyelitis (CDEM). These syndromes result in multiple sclerosis-like symptoms of paralysis, weakness, tingling, numbness, pain, and cognitive deficit. As a result, some people have to be put on a ventilator to assist with breathing. There is no cure for GBS or other demyelinating syndromes, and the health issues associated with these conditions can last anywhere from three to four weeks to a lifetime. These syndromes can appear anywhere from twenty-four hours up to six weeks after vaccination, and many healthcare providers are reluctant to report them to VAERS; even worse, healthcare providers may not even know about VAERS, despite federal requirements for reporting adverse reactions to the database.

MYTH #4: ONCE YOU GET VACCINATED FOR INFLUENZA, YOU ARE PROTECTED RIGHT AWAY FROM GETTING INFLUENZA FOR THE REST OF THE FLU SEASON.

Many of the patients I've talked to think that they're protected against influenza as soon as they get the shot. They also think they can't get influenza for the rest of the season.

The CDC itself tells people that it takes at least two weeks to build up antibodies against influenza after receiving the vaccine. This is a big assumption — not everyone's immune system is able to muster a response against viruses, for various reasons ranging from immuno-suppression therapy to even just being in a bad mood when getting the vaccine.[184] Moreover, immunity can wane over the course of the season. This partially explains why we often see surges of influenza in March, when the vaccine might no longer be effective in a person who was vaccinated in September.

MYTH #5: YOU CAN'T GET INFLUENZA FROM THE VACCINE.

Technically speaking, this one is sort of true, although the risk of bias and lack of statistical significance in studies makes it difficult to sort out fact from myth. What you can definitely get from the vaccine are influenza-like symptoms — fever, malaise, stuffy nose, etc. — that are caused by your immune system asking, "What the heck did you just inject into me?" This happens most frequently when the vaccine is given at the same time as other vaccines, such as the pneumococcal vaccine. The CDC recommends that children do not receive the influenza and pneumococcal vaccines at the same time due to the increased risk of febrile seizures.[185] Yet these vaccines in fact are often administered together — another reason to question the safety studies and the education of people giving the vaccines!

Because of its toxic ingredients, the influenza vaccine also weakens your immune system for an unspecified amount of time after vaccination, possibly making you more susceptible to other circulating viruses such as rhinovirus, which causes the common cold. During the 2009 H1N1 "pandemic," people who received the inactivated influenza vaccine, which did not contain H1N1, were more likely to be hospitalized with complications attributed to H1N1 infection.[186]

MYTH #6: YOU CAN'T GIVE SOMEONE ELSE INFLUENZA IF YOU'VE BEEN VACCINATED

People who receive the live attenuated influenza vaccine (LAIV) can transmit influenza to people up to three weeks after vaccination, especially to those who are immunocompromised, i.e., on medications such as steroids and/or chemotherapy.[187] High rates of vaccine failure mean that people who get the influenza vaccine could still be susceptible to influenza infection. Then they can transmit influenza or an influenza-like virus while contagious. Remember how the CDC had to change its definition of "efficiency" in Myth #2?

MYTH #7: VACCINATION IS THE ONLY WAY TO PREVENT INFLUENZA.

Much of the dogma surrounding influenza and other vaccine policies is based on the theory of herd immunity: the idea that if enough people in "the herd" get vaccinated, then the virus can't spread and will die out. No scientific studies have ever proven this hypothesis in any laboratory or real-life setting, but many public health policies are based on it anyway. Unfortunately, viruses are smart little strands of genetic codes that can mutate and differentiate in order to survive, despite our best intentions.[188]

It is illogical to rely on vaccination as the sole method of disease prevention. We have to use common sense and all of the tools that nature gives us. You have the power to both strengthen your immune system against influenza and prevent influenza transmission to others, with or without a vaccine. Here are nine easy and beneficial habits to adopt.

1. Hand hygiene. Handwashing is truly the most understated public health measure that you can take to keep yourself and others healthy (assuming that you have access to clean water). Sing "Twinkle, Twinkle, Little Star" or "Happy Birthday" twice through with your kids to make sure everyone has washed long enough.

2. Cover your mouth! Just not with your hand. Cough and sneeze into your sleeve, please. This is not one hundred percent preventative, but it can help to stop thousands of virus-containing droplets from shooting everywhere with each cough and sneeze.

3. Don't pick your nose or bite your fingernails. Picking your nose is one of the fastest and easiest ways to introduce the influenza virus into your body. If you must get that booger out, use a tissue. Same thing goes for biting your fingernails because of the bacteria and viruses lurking underneath. If you haven't recently washed your hands, sticking your fingers in your mouth

during flu season is a bad idea. Find another habit, such as using a stress ball or taking sips of water, to keep your hands and mouth happy in those stressful or boring situations.

4. Reduce sugar and carbohydrate consumption. Sugars and empty carbs (like white bread, pasta, and French fries) deplete the immune system on many levels. First, they rob your immune system of important nutrients, especially minerals like calcium and magnesium, needed to ward off invasion from viruses like influenza. They also raise insulin levels in the blood, which can prevent the immune system from doing its job of stopping viral invaders.[189] Sugars and empty carbs can also quickly damage the microbiome in your digestive system, where eighty percent of your immune system resides in the mucosa-associated lymphoid tissue (MALT). Instead, fill your diet with fresh vegetables, complete proteins from organic, sustainably-sourced animals and legumes, and healthy fats such as butter, coconut oil, avocado, and extra-virgin olive oil. I dream of how many people would benefit from the removal of sodas, sweetened beverages, and empty carbs from hospital cafeterias and patient trays, especially during "flu season."

5. Feed your microbiome. Why is the microbiome such a popular topic of discussion in healthcare these days? Because the health of our own cells depends on the health of our microbiome: the symbiotic bacteria, fungi, yeasts, and helminths that live inside and on us. Feeding your microbiome means not only consuming foods rich in probiotics but also consuming foods that nourish the environment of your gastrointestinal (GI) tract so the microbiome can flourish. Raw fermented sauerkraut is truly a superfood because it is rich in vitamin C (which is why sailors of the old navies would bring barrels of it on their voyages), fiber, and health-nourishing bacteria, all of which keep your immune system ready for battle. Other options to feed your microbiome include kale, whole-milk plain yogurt, kefir, kombucha, and apple cider vinegar. Please consult with your holistic healthcare provider before purchasing an over-the-counter probiotic to make sure you are getting what you

need. Remember that many pharmaceutical drugs — including vaccines but especially steroids and antibiotics — can harm the health of your microbiome, so be sure to talk with your prescriber about this issue before starting any medications.

6. Get a good night's sleep, at least seven to eight hours daily. How often have you felt like you were coming down with something, only to stave it off with a good night's sleep? Our ancestors were smart to sleep with the darkness of winter, because sleep is when the healing magic happens. Sleep deprivation puts your immune system to sleep.[190] If we get enough sleep, we give ourselves an advantage when it comes to beating the flu.

7. Keep your child home from school if they say they don't feel well or if they have a fever. I realize that some companies and schools have more generous sick leave policies than others, but staying home when sick — quarantining yourself or a sick child — is the right thing to do when it comes to stopping virus transmission. Staying home can also allow your child time to rest and sleep so that their immune system can go to work on getting them well again.

8. Get fresh air. One of the reasons people tend to get sick in the winter is because they are in close quarters with each other in stale air. Unless it's dangerously cold out, bundle up the kids and let them play outside each day. You can go outside, too!

9. Consult with a trained holistic healthcare provider to learn ways to strengthen your immune system, microbiome, and general health with whole food nutrients and herbs. Not all products are created equal! Self-prescribing can often take us down a more expensive rabbit hole than the cost of a consultation, so it's worth spending a little extra money on someone who understands how nutrients and herbs impact the body. I don't recommend going it alone and buying products willy-nilly. Spend the time and money working with someone who understands your health and your needs.

Research, educate, and empower yourself by reading books and independent research articles (such as those found at greenmedinfo. com). Then make an informed decision about what is right for you and your family.

Whatever you decide about vaccines, make sure that it's a decision you feel good about and that you don't feel coerced, forced, or frightened into doing something against your will. It's easy to get upset when discussing these issues; instead, channel your frustration into action by doing your homework first. Empowering ourselves with knowledge is the first step on the road to natural wellness and healing for good.

10

VACCINE RECOVERY

By Brittany Love

"Nature is our ultimate healer."

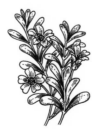

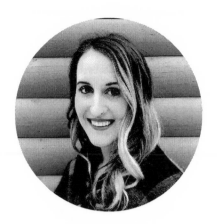

Brittany Love is a mother of three who resides outside Baltimore, Maryland. She is a successful entrepreneur who combines her training in early childhood education and birth and doula work with her passion for all things natural health. She is a certified Psych K practitioner who has assisted many in healing from the inside out. Her children are her greatest sources of joy, and she is blessed to both homeschool them and teach at their classical co-op. In her spare time, Brittany enjoys making flower essences, using essential oils, and promoting a message of hope for those struggling with various health issues.

ig: @b.love.healing

Before I share my story, I think it's important for you to understand the difference in my life before and after my vaccine injury.

I grew up in Baltimore, Maryland with my parents and brother. I spent my childhood running barefoot outside, crabbing on the Chesapeake Bay with my grandpa, and babysitting for all the neighborhood kids. I was active and healthy. By the age of five, I had received about eight vaccines with no noticeable reactions. As I got older, I decided to work with children and dreamed of living abroad and working with orphans in developing countries. In pursuit of my dreams, I traveled to Europe and Central America and worked in orphanages.

My travels came to a halt when I received the HPV vaccine at the age of twenty. This is where my story begins. Until that point, I was vibrant and healthy, but all that changed the day I received the vaccine. I was to be married and so I set up my first OB-GYN appointment. I was a virgin at the time and had never had a Pap smear. The day of my office visit, I was nervous but excited for what my future held. I wanted lots of children, and my partner and I planned to have kids soon after we got married.

I had no idea that one visit to the doctor would change the entire course of my life. The HPV vaccine was fairly new and not much was known about it. My doctor told me that it prevented cervical cancer. No side effects were explained to me; she never gave me a package insert or additional information. In fact, there was no mention of HPV itself.

I received the first round of shots that day and within hours, the worst flu of my life came over me. I became extremely dizzy — a dizziness that would last for the next ten years. The fatigue was so crippling that I couldn't stay awake, and my entire body hurt. I slept and slept. When I was awake, I experienced horrible brain fog, pain, and dizziness.

After about a week, I began functioning again but I was very slow compared to before the shot. In fact, I was never the same. I continued to experience terrible brain fog, body pain, dizziness, memory issues, motion sickness, allergies, depression, and a general unwell feeling.

When I went back to my doctor for the second round of shots, I explained to her what had happened. She told me this was a normal reaction and that after the third and last shot, my body would work itself out and I'd feel better. I believed her, thinking that my reaction was normal and that all symptoms would go away once I'd completed the series. Every part of my being was screaming, "No!," but I got the second shot that day.

All of my symptoms escalated, and I developed even worse symptoms. I had to wear a heart monitor because my heart skipped so much. I was so dizzy that I felt faint all the time. Nausea was now a regular occurrence, and I developed many food allergies. I also developed irritable bowel syndrome and lost so much weight that I fell into the underweight category. I was five-foot-eight and weighed only one hundred and fifteen pounds. I became a shell of the woman I once knew.

Back then, nobody I knew who had received the HPV vaccine reacted this way. As it later turned out, thousands of patients had an experience similar to mine, but I wouldn't meet them and hear their story until years later.

We now know that HPV vaccines have caused thousands of adverse reactions,[195] including reports of sudden collapse with unconsciousness within twenty-four hours, seizures, muscle pain and weakness, disabling fatigue, Guillain Barre Syndrome (GBS), facial paralysis, brain inflammation, rheumatoid arthritis, lupus, blood clots, optic neuritis, multiple sclerosis, strokes, and heart and other serious health problems, including death.[196]

Those of us who received the vaccine in the early days did not understand the dangers; many of us were not informed by our doctors or nurses. I count myself lucky because many girls aren't here to tell their stories. Sadly, this vaccine has stolen many healthy lives.

About a year after I received the HPV vaccine, when I was thirty-two weeks pregnant with my first son, my doctors diagnosed me with lupus, an autoimmune disease. The entire pregnancy was rough for me, but knowing what I know now, I count myself blessed to have gotten pregnant at all.

During my pregnancy, I received two additional vaccines: the flu shot and the H1N1 shot. Shortly after these shots, I became hospitalized. I lived on hospital bed rest from thirty to thirty-two weeks with a condition known as lupus-induced preeclampsia. My sweet little baby was born prematurely by emergency cesarean section. He weighed only two pounds, fourteen ounces. He is my miracle boy.

Sadly, I assumed that only the newer vaccines on the market were causing issues, and I vaccinated my son with all the traditional vaccines. He had two separate reactions, one of which landed him in the hospital. He developed anaphylactic allergies, eczema, and high-functioning autism.

I hope to share what I have learned with you to spare you the years I lost. It's been eleven years since my life changed so drastically, and although I'm not running any marathons yet, in many ways I have healed my body and gotten my life back.

I began my natural healing journey soon after my son's second vaccine reaction. I walked away from Western medicine and found solace and hope in the natural healing world. We worked with a naturopath and a homeopathic doctor to get our lives back. It was a ten-year journey for me and a seven-year journey for my son. Through the use of healing foods, natural supplements, essential oils, redox signaling molecules, chiropractic care, acupuncture, and lots of deep soul work, my son and I have been able to mostly recover our lives.

Healing foods played such a crucial role in our journey. We cut out inflammatory foods (gluten and dairy) and mainly stuck to a plant-based diet low in meat. Fruits also formed a huge part of our healing, and juicing and smoothies became a part of our daily lives. We switched all of our vitamins and supplements to ones that are plant-based and made of whole foods. We chose organic everything and were careful what we put into our bodies.

Our home also became chemical-free; we use essential oils for almost everything. We clean with them, and we even use them for tummy aches and flus.

Although we came so far using our natural remedies, our bodies were still struggling to detox and heal. It was a slow-going process, and I prayed for something that would speed up our healing. Then I discovered redox signaling molecules. I can say with certainty that these molecules helped us like nothing had before. Redox signaling molecules help the cells to renew, repair, and regenerate. These molecules are native to the body and help upregulate the body's own glutathione by over five hundred percent. Glutathione is an antioxidant commonly found in animals, plants, fungi, and bacteria that help neutralize free radicals and prevent cellular damage.[197] For proper functioning of our body, we need oxygen, water, glucose, andl glutathione molecules in limited proportions. Together, all these molecules are the backbone of energy production in our body.

Genetic studies have shown that redox signaling molecules play key roles in the body's detox pathways. When we began supplementing with these molecules, we noticed quickly how different we felt. The brain fog lifted, my dizziness decreased and eventually went away, and we slept great and woke up energized. We began feeling healthy and vibrant. Two and a half years later, we are still using these amazing molecules, and I don't think we'd be where we are without them. They provided what our bodies needed to heal themselves.

I also need to mention the inner healing aspect of recovery. Natural healing looks at the whole person, not just the physical symptoms. We did lots of energy work to heal from the inside out. We practice Psych-K, Bodytalk, EFT, AFT, reiki, NET, and lots of talk therapy. Inner healing is so important when you're trying to heal your body of dis-ease. My spirituality and healing of my heart and soul were equally, if not more, important as the healing of my body. As I healed on the inside and made peace with God, my physical body caught up. We are not separate from our souls. I think many people miss out on healing because they only look at the physical and neglect what's more important — healing the heart.

My son is no longer diagnosed with autism, and my lupus labs look so clean that I don't even appear to have the disease now. As there is no known cure for lupus, I count this as a miracle.

There was so much I didn't know about vaccines, especially the HPV vaccine. We now know that the HPV vaccine has the highest rate of adverse reactions; many countries have pulled the vaccine off the market and many doctors have spoken out against it. Dr. Harper, one of the developers of the vaccine, has repeatedly spoken out against it and has concerns regarding whether or not the vaccine is safe.[198] In Japan, the vaccine was taken off the market after many young girls showed adverse reactions.[199] The same thing happened in a small village in Colombia, where many young girls became very ill after receiving the HPV vaccine.[200] Ireland has issued warnings and has seen court cases fighting for those injured by this horrific vaccine.[201]

Furthermore, we know that the type of HPV that causes cervical cancer is extremely slow-growing and that the best protection against it is regular Pap screenings. All in all, the risks of the HPV vaccine seem to far outweigh any of its originally intended benefits.

I returned to my doctor months later and was offered the third and final shot in the series. I said no. A few months after receiving my second dose, I had found a chiropractor who informed me of the risks of the vaccine and began working to reverse the damage as much as he could. When I confidently refused the third shot, my doctor got upset. I ended up walking out of her office. She never reported my reactions or believed my symptoms stemmed from the vaccine. I do not know if she feels differently now, as I never went back to her and have not seen or spoken to her since.

These days, I'm continuing with my healing journey one step at a time as I enjoy raising my beautiful children. We spend our days in nature, soaking up all the healing it has to offer.

I share my story in the hopes that if I can help one person not endure the decade of suffering that I did, then I'll have done some good in the world. I wish I knew then what I know now, but that knowledge is what I hope to pass on. If I could go back and tell my younger self one thing, it would be to trust my instincts more. Read the package inserts and do the research for yourself. Trust in your body's amazing healing abilities and know that God provided us with astounding things on the Earth to keep us healthy and thriving. Nature is our ultimate healer.

11

YOU ARE WHAT YOU INJECT

By Noemi Elizabeth Hermling

"You are what you eat.
You are what you inject."

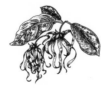

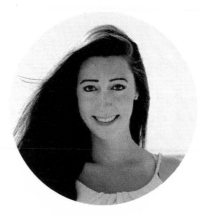

Noemi Elizabeth Hermling is a twenty-seven-year-old mother of two and certified vaccine education specialist. She has spent her life traveling the globe, absorbing and immersing herself in the cultures around her. She reveals her enthusiastic and persuasive personality through her work as an activist and social media influencer, using her platform to educate her followers on human trafficking, vaccination safety and efficacy, and natural parenting. She is currently pursuing her nursing degree and aspires to land a job as a registered nurse in a Newborn Intensive Care Unit. She holds two citizenships, one in the United States and the other in Spain, and is bilingual, speaking both English and Castilian fluently. Her discipline is deep-rooted after years as a competitive figure skater, concert pianist, and volleyball player, and she continues to hone her skills in each of these areas. She also enjoys sewing, world travel, and open water diving. She believes that her faith is stronger than her fears and that the truth must always be shared, regardless of the ramifications. As Mahatma Gandhi said, "Truth never damages a cause that is just."

fb: @noemi.hermling | ig: @noemielizabethofficial

There is an old saying: "You are what you eat." In my home, we check food labels, scouring the laundry list of ingredients for chemicals and additives that could potentially be harmful and toxic to our children. After all, as parents, it is our responsibility to investigate what our children are consuming and coming into contact with. If you were given a beverage that contained toxic, carcinogenic ingredients, would you drink it? Would you give it to your children?

What if these same ingredients were injected right into your child's bloodstream?

At a minimum, parents should be informed. This extends beyond controversy. This is more than just a needle prick.

The problems with routine vaccination highlight the fact that we have been misled into believing that toxicities aren't harmful when they come in injected form. Perhaps we've conditioned ourselves into believing physicians and their immunization recommendations despite the inadequate professional education they have received on critical vaccine safety and efficacy. Perhaps we are afraid of the diseases that vaccines claim to protect our children from.

Whatever the case may be, as parents, it is our right to express our concerns and our duty to investigate absolutely everything we give our children. We have the tools to research and the aptitude to study vaccine manufacturer inserts. We are not exempt from learning about vaccinations and their ingredients or from evaluating their safety and efficacy prior to making any permanent medical decisions.

As of 2018, the Center for Disease Control recommends seventy-two individual doses of vaccines from birth to age eighteen, including the annual flu shot.[202] The number of available vaccines has since increased due to the recent approval of the anthrax vaccine, Japanese encephalitis vaccine, and haxavalent vaccine. It doesn't stop there. As of 2016, nearly three hundred vaccinations were in the pipeline awaiting approval in the United States.[203] Each individual manufacturer's vaccine insert is available on the Center for Disease Control (CDC) website or at your nearest vaccine-administering clinic. It's important to note that the Vaccine Information Sheet provided by your doctor is not the manufacturer insert and does not include specific vaccine ingredient information or post-marketing effects. The manufacturer insert is extensively detailed, pages long, and comes tightly folded in the original vaccine manufacturer's box. This is required by law.

Most vaccines have "not been evaluated for their mutagenic and carcinogenic effects," as stated on several vaccine manufacturer inserts, including the Pertussis and MMR Vaccine Insert. This leads me to question how we can administer a vaccine to our children without proof that the ingredients within these vaccines are not damaging the most vulnerable people on Earth. Children are the leaders of our future generations, and it is our duty as parents to make informed and educated decisions on their behalf. The Center for Disease Control Vaccine Excipient and Media Summary is a great place to start your research. This document is available on the CDC website and contains a detailed list of ingredients extracted from each vaccine report.

The following information may be difficult to digest. Two of the most controversial vaccine ingredients you will find listed throughout the Excipient and Media Summary are MRC-5 and WI-38 human diploid lung fibroblasts. WI-38 is a diploid human cell strain derived from the lung tissue of an aborted three-month gestation female. MRC-5 is a diploid human cell strain derived from the lung tissue of an aborted fourteen-week gestation male.

The effects of injecting foreign DNA and cell cultures from aborted babies have not been tested by the CDC or FDA. However, several independent studies have evaluated the biological effects of vaccine contaminants and the correlative Autism Spectrum Disorder (ASD) diagnosis change-points. An in-depth analysis done by Theresa Deisher, Ph.D. confirmed the autism change-points in children and correlative data that exposed the biological effects of vaccine contaminants.[204] The data was consistent with the incline of ASD diagnosis since the introduction of foreign DNA in vaccinations.

The recommended childhood vaccines that contain either MRC-5 or WI-38 cell strains, or both, are DTaP-IPV, DTaP-IPV/Hib, hepatitis A, hepatitis A/hepatitis B, MMR, MMRV, and varicella.[205]

Nearly all vaccinations contain cells derived from human aborted fetal tissue, such as MRC-5 and WI-38, canine cells (such as MDCK), monkey cells (referred to as VERO cells), or chicken cells derived from chick embryos.

A genetic therapy analysis concluded that four out of nine boys who were given essentially the same ingredients as the contaminants in vaccines (human DNA fragments and MMLV retrovirus fragments) developed cancer, specifically leukemia.[206]

Time trends compiled from three ongoing data sets, including the California Department of Developmental Services, Individuals with Disabilities Education Act, and Autism and Developmental Disabilities Monitoring Network, confirm the steadily rapid rate of increase for Autism Spectrum Disorder diagnoses in children between the years 1930 and 2014.

Human diploid cells are just the tip of the iceberg when it comes to exposing vaccine ingredients and their inadequate pre-marketing testing for safety.

Formaldehyde has been found in popular cereal brands and has sparked outrage from parents who unknowingly fed their children a toxic breakfast that contained a cancer-causing ingredient. The International Agency for Research on Cancer has concluded that formaldehyde, which is present in herbicides, pesticides, building materials, and embalming fluid, is carcinogenic in humans.[207] Formaldehyde is used in vaccines to inactivate the virus so the person being inoculated does not contract the disease. Formalin, formaldehyde in water, plays a prevalent role in several recommended childhood vaccinations, such as DT, DTap, DTap-IPV, DTaP-HepB-IPV, DTaP-IPV/Hib, Hib, hepatitis A, hepatitis B, influenza, meningococcal, polio, and TDaP.[208]

A quick search through the vaccine manufacturer inserts will reveal that several vaccines containing formaldehyde, including but not limited to TDaP, "have not been evaluated for carcinogenic or mutagenic potential, or for impairment of fertility."[209]

At just a few hours old, our newborns are injected with the hepatitis B vaccination, even if the birth mother has been confirmed as hepatitis B-negative through routine prenatal blood work. Forms of the hepatitis B vaccine are contaminated with formaldehyde, among other toxicities, and the vaccine's adverse effects are extensive, including but not limited to anaphylactic reactions, eczema, Guillain-Barré syndrome, optic neuritis, arthritis, thrombocytopenia, syncope, and tachycardia.[210]

The Food and Drug Administration approves these vaccinations, which get injected into our youth despite hundreds of adverse effects reported during the vaccine's post-marketing period.

Picking through the extensive listing of vaccine ingredients provided by the CDC, we see neomycin, aluminum, fetal bovine serum, polysorbate 80, VERO cells, yeast and egg protein, and thimerosal (mercury). Neomycin is a known carcinogen, used in vaccines during the production and storage stages to prevent the growth of bacteria.

Aluminum, also a known carcinogen and neurotoxin, is used as an adjuvant to help the vaccine work more quickly. Aluminum is capable of destroying the neurons necessary for cognitive and motor functions; children in developed nations are exposed to significant amounts of aluminum in vaccines. These repeated exposures with multi-dose vaccines during critical periods of neurodevelopment can provoke permanent malfunctions of the brain and immune system.[211]

Babies who follow the recommended immunization schedule are exposed to 4,925 mcg (4.9mg) of aluminum by eighteen months of age. This level has not been evaluated for safety in children, nor have the effects of aluminum exposure via injection during crucial neurodevelopmental periods.

A simplified way to understand the effects of ingestion versus injection is to have one individual consume three shots of tequila and to inject another individual with three shots of the same liquor. It's known that the bodily response to alcohol injected into the bloodstream is going to be much more severe and detrimental.

Fetal bovine serum provides cells the optimum nutrition to grow viruses in the laboratory. However, collecting fetal bovine serum is far from humane. No anesthesia is given to fetal calves when their heart is punctured between the ribs, and blood is withdrawn for several minutes. It's estimated that fetal calves can remain alive for up to thirty minutes post-collection. Several studies suggest there is a possibility that serum can be contaminated with viruses, bacteria, mycoplasmas, yeast, fungi, immunoglobulins, endotoxins, and possibly prions, with the potential to induce fatal neurodegenerative diseases. MMR, DTaP, polio, hepatitis A, rotavirus, Japanese encephalitis, and varicella vaccines all contain fetal bovine serum or bovine extracts.[212]

Polysorbate 80 is used as an excipient, essentially thickening the vaccine for proper dosage, and as an emulsifier to bond the ingredients. Upon injection, polysorbate 80 opens the blood-brain barrier, allowing toxins to enter the brain. DTaP, DTaP-IPV, DTaP-HepB-IPV, DTaP-IPV/Hib, hepatitis A, hepatitis B, hepatitis A/hepatitis B, HPV, influenza, meningococcal, pneumococcal, rotavirus, and TDaP vaccines all contain polysorbate 80.[213]

African Green Monkey cells, otherwise known as VERO cells, are derived from the kidney of an adult African Green Monkey and are present in DTaP-IPV, DTaP-HepB-IPV, polio, rotavirus, and smallpox vaccines. If your child is allergic to dairy, eggs, or soy, they should not receive any of the vaccinations that contain these proteins due to the risk of severe allergic or hypersensitivity reactions, including anaphylaxis. The vaccines containing one or more of these proteins are the influenza vaccine, DTaP-HepB-IPV, hepatitis A/hepatitis B, HPV, hepatitis B, meningococcal, and pneumococcal.

Thimerosal, which contains mercury, is an organomercury compound used as a preservative in multi-dose vials when more than one needle is inserted into the vial. Considerations and studies on this additive have not been performed by the Center for Disease Control or Food and Drug Administration. However, until 2002, high quantities of thimerosal were present in the TDaP, hepatitis B, and Hib vaccines. Thimerosal is still present in influenza vaccines, which are given to pregnant women, infants, and children. Why is thimerosal still present in the influenza vaccines, you might ask? The World Health Organization estimated that manufacturing multi-dose (ten-dose) vials saves approximately fifteen cents per vaccine dose compared to single-dose vials without thimerosal (mercury).[214]

If your child accidentally consumed a bottle of aluminum, formaldehyde, fetal bovine serum, human diploid cells, neomycin, chick embryo cell cultures, thimerosal, and African Green Monkey kidney cells, you would be advised to call Poison Control immediately and take them to the emergency room to be evaluated for toxic exposures. The measles, mumps, and rubella vaccine (MMR) is a live attenuated virus. That means that upon injection, your child can actually contract a measles rash, mumps, or rubella. This also means that for up to six weeks post-vaccination, your child can shed the live virus to immunocompromised individuals, newborn babies, and pregnant women. Vaccinated children are also susceptible to contracting measles, mumps, and rubella due to the vaccines efficacy rate. The same is true for the live influenza vaccine, varicella vaccine, and pertussis (whooping cough) vaccine. After receiving the pertussis vaccine, an individual can be an asymptomatic carrier and shed whooping cough onto newborn babies who cannot be immunized against pertussis.

The ingredients in vaccines are directly responsible for thousands of vaccine injuries and deaths reported to VAERS, the Vaccine Adverse Event Reporting System. The Vaccine Injury Compensation Program has awarded over four billion U.S. dollars to the victims of vaccine injury and to the families of those who have died as a result of vaccination, with a cap of two hundred and fifty thousand dollars per case.[215 216] Vaccinations directly affect the neurodevelopment of our children, and it's particularly concerning that the toxicities present in vaccines have not been evaluated for their carcinogenic and mutagenic potential. The 2013 Childhood Immunization Schedule and Safety Publication by the Institute of Medicine's Committee on the Assessment of Studies of Health Outcomes Related to the Recommended Childhood Immunization Schedule concluded that "studies designed to examine the long-term effects of the cumulative number of vaccines or other aspects of the immunization schedule have not been conducted."[217]

While vaccine injuries and death may not occur in every child, no child is exempt from suffering at the hands of the vaccine industry. As the vaccine industry expands, so will the reported adverse effects from these unsupported, non-tested, and biased immunization recommendations. Every child is uniquely different, from their genetics and their microbiome to their health history. Each child will react to vaccines differently. However, regardless of how small a quantity of these toxic ingredients is included in vaccines, the fact remains that they have not been tested adequately. That is the biggest point of concern.

The comprehensive, peer-reviewed scientific studies on vaccine ingredients such as thimerosal, mercury, aluminum adjuvants, and other toxicities cannot be overlooked. Vaccine makers stand to make billions at the hands of our children and their health. Vaccinations are unfortunately not as clear cut as one would assume. Based upon the facts I have given you, I encourage you to do your own research and find a licensed physician who you trust with your child's health. Where there is a risk, there must always be a choice, and where there is a choice, there must always be an educated, fully informed decision. Our children deserve it.

12

AWAKENING: 'DEADLY' DISEASES BY THE NUMBERS

By Meghan Rose

"By educating one person at a time, we can empower people to make informed decisions that they are 100% confident in, and take back our children's health and future."

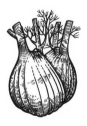

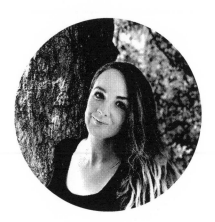

Meghan Rose is a retired infectious disease registered nurse who is sickened by the acceptance of chronic childhood illness as the new normal. She believes that we are created perfectly and that true health does not come from pharmaceuticals. Meghan is passionate about educating and empowering parents to be one hundred percent confident in the decisions they make regarding their children's health through their own research, and she has worked with hundreds of people who have healed their bodies through natural means. Meghan lives in the United States with her husband and six children. She is a certified vaccine education specialist and global online entrepreneur.

ig: @MeghanRoseOfficial | fb: MeghanRose

I had always been very "by the book" when it comes to medical treatment and prevention, especially when it came to vaccines. I never had any reason to question their safety or effectiveness and always believed that "anti-vaxxers" had to be either crazy or uneducated. The first time I ever gave thought to the idea that vaccines could potentially be harmful was while I was working as a school nurse. Out of a total student body of about six hundred students, only two children had vaccine exemptions, one of them being from a family whose baby had passed away following his six month shots. Even then . . . I was convinced that this had to be a one-in-a-million incident.

Working in the elementary school was eye-opening. I soon learned that our children are just not as healthy as they were when I was growing up. The change was not only dramatic, it was alarming: food allergies, asthma, learning disabilities, diabetes, seizure disorders, entire classrooms dedicated to children on the autism spectrum. Times have definitely changed, and it wasn't until this health crisis hit close to home that my eyes became truly opened to the scale of it.

One of my sons started to struggle with extreme hyperactivity. I brushed it off at first, thinking it was normal "boy" behavior. However, it got to the point where every single year, with every single teacher, I was hearing the same story. My son just could not function in class. He literally could not sit still; he struggled with boundaries and verbal outbursts and often ended up isolated from the rest of the classroom. It killed me inside to think about medicating my son, but in the end, I didn't think it was fair to him to continue to put him through the trouble at school. I finally brought him to his pediatrician for help and he was prescribed ADHD medication.

The medication "worked" at first. We received great reports from my son's teachers about how calm he was, and on a couple of occasions when we missed doses, I would get negative reports home. After a few months, though, the effects started to wear off altogether and we had to increase the dosage.

Not too soon after, the side effects started. First, my son lost his appetite and had terrible trouble sleeping. Then he became zombie-like, losing all expression of emotion. After a few months, the positive effects of the medication again wore off but the negative effects continued. Again, his pediatrician increased the dose, and again, after a few months, the positive effects wore off while the negative side effects continued to get worse.

My son didn't want to eat at all, he wasn't sleeping, and then one day, he started to experience heart palpitations. I was scared. I read over all of the side effects and thought to myself, "This is absolutely crazy to have him on this medication that could potentially kill him — just so he would be more calm?" There had to be a better way, and that was the first time in my life that I entertained the idea of natural health remedies.

We put my son on an autoimmune diet along with a few natural supplements, and within just one week, we started to see a huge change. He was experiencing all of the positive, calming effects that he had with his medication without being a complete zombie and without the negative side effects. It was incredible. I fervently started researching all things natural and holistic. We changed our diet to completely organic and cut out most of the toxic chemicals that we were using on our bodies and in our cleaning products . . . but we were still vaccinating.

And then I really woke up.

In 2016, there was an enormous media stink over a new documentary, *VAXXED*. The movie suddenly got pulled from a film festival before ever being shown. I would probably never have watched it if it hadn't been pulled, but boy, am I glad that it was. Because there was such an urgency to suppress the information, I had to know the motive behind the decision.

That documentary blew me away. It did not talk about vaccines themselves and why parents shouldn't use them; there was no trying to convince any parents of anything like that. Rather, the documentary covered a senior Centers for Disease Control scientist who blew the whistle about how the CDC disposed of information showing that African American boys were at a significantly higher risk of developing autism if they received the MMR vaccine when given on time per the recommended schedule. I just could not believe that this had happened, and I could not understand how nothing had changed in the almost fifteen years since they initially performed the study. It was angering. I had to learn more.

I had heard previously that vaccines were not responsible for the decline in deaths from infectious disease, but being a nurse and pro-vaccine, I always dismissed this finding as ridiculous. Now I went in search of the real numbers.

I wanted to know the death rates from infectious diseases before the introduction of vaccines versus the numbers after. What exactly are these "diseases"? What is my risk of infection? Are they treatable? If yes, how so? What is the risk of infection? What are the symptoms? What are the case-mortality rates? You know . . . the actual *facts*. Because when significant amounts of money are involved, science can be skewed. We call this tobacco science.

So here, I would like to present you with just that — the facts, summarized, according to the CDC.

DIPHTHERIA

What is it? Diphtheria is a bacterial disease caused by the bacterium *Corynebacterium diphtheriae*. The disease typically spreads through respiratory droplets produced by coughing or sneezing but also can be transmitted when a person comes into contact with an object that has the bacteria on it. Symptoms include weakness, sore throat, fever, and swollen neck glands.

Risk of infection: During the 1920s, before the introduction of the diphtheria vaccination, the risk of catching diphtheria was about one hundred and fifty per one hundred thousand people (0.15 percent of population). Today, diphtheria is still a rare disease in industrialized countries, with only five cases reported since 2000.

Overall case-fatality rate: The fatality rate for diphtheria is between five and ten percent, with higher death rates (up to twenty percent) among children younger than five years old and adults older than forty.

Treatability: Diphtheria can be treated with antibiotics. In research conducted in 1934-1935, Dr. Fred Klenner and other physicians also discovered that vitamin C (ascorbic acid) can be used to treat the disease.

HAEMOPHILUS INFLUENZAE TYPE B (HIB)

What is it? Haemophilus influenzae type b, or Hib, is a bacterial infection that occurs most commonly in young children. The disease typically spreads through respiratory droplets produced from coughing or sneezing. There are varying types of infections caused by the disease, and symptoms depend on the area of the body infected:

- Pneumonia: fever and chills, cough, shortness of breath, sweating, chest pain, headache, muscle pain or aches, and excessive tiredness
- Bacteremia: fever and chills, excessive tiredness, belly pain, nausea, diarrhea, anxiety, and altered mental status
- Meningitis: fever, headache, stiff neck, nausea, photophobia (eye discomfort or pain), and altered mental status

Risk of infection: Hib is not common in the United States. The disease occurs primarily among children younger than five years of age. In the pre-vaccine era, the highest incidence rate was 0.19% in the six- to seven-year-old age range. All other age ranges had lower incidence rate.

Overall case-fatality rate: For children infected with the disease, between three and six percent of Hib cases are fatal. Patients aged sixty-five years and older have higher case-fatality ratios than children.

Treatability: Hib can be treated with antibiotics; in some cases, patients may need breathing treatments.

HEPATITIS A

What is it? Hepatitis A is a viral infection of the liver. People typically acquire the disease by ingesting food, drinks, or objects contaminated by small, undetected amounts of stool from an infected person (otherwise known as the fecal-oral route); hepatitis A can also spread from close personal contact with an infected person, such as through sex or caring for someone who is ill. Hepatitis A is usually a short-term infection and does not become chronic. Symptoms include fever, malaise, anorexia, nausea, abdominal discomfort, dark urine, and jaundice.

Risk of infection: In the early to mid-1990s, among children ages two to eighteen years, there were between fifteen and twenty cases of hepatitis A per one hundred thousand children (0.02 percent of the population). In 2016, there were an estimated four thousand total hepatitis A cases in the United States.

Overall case-fatality rate: Among all reported cases (persons of all ages), the fatality rate for hepatitis A was approximately 0.3 percent. For patients aged forty years or more, the fatality rate may have been around two percent.

Treatability: Symptomatic management includes rest, adequate nutrition, and fluids.

HEPATITIS B

What is it? Hepatitis B is a liver infection caused by the hepatitis B virus (HBV). The disease spreads when blood, semen, or other bodily fluid from a person infected with the hepatitis B virus enters the body of someone who is not infected: for example, through sexual contact, sharing needles or syringes, or at birth from mother to baby. Symptoms include fever, fatigue, loss of appetite, nausea, vomiting, abdominal pain, dark urine, clay-colored bowel movements, joint pain, and jaundice.

Risk of infection: In the mid-1980s, there were about twenty-six thousand cases reported each year in the United States; in 1996, this rate fell below ten thousand cases (0.003 percent of the population).

Overall case-mortality rate: In 2008, the mortality rate for hepatitis B was 0.5 deaths per one hundred thousand people (0.0005 percent of the population).

Treatability: There is no treatment for acute hepatitis B, but rest, adequate nutrition, and fluids are recommended to manage symptoms.

MEASLES

What is it? Measles is an acute viral infection spread through the air from coughing or sneezing. The disease can also spread if people touch an infected surface and then touch their eyes, noses, or mouths. Symptoms include fever, runny nose, cough, red eyes, and sore throat, followed by a rash that spreads over the body.

Risk of infection: Before the introduction of the vaccination in 1963, approximately five hundred thousand cases of measles were reported annually in the United States; it was considered a childhood rite-of-passage, as common as the common cold. More than fifty percent of persons had measles by age six, and more than ninety percent had measles by age fifteen.

Overall case-mortality rate: Before the introduction of the vaccine, the case-mortality rate for measles was 0.2 percent.

Treatability: In an article published in Cochrane Review, authors of a study involving 2,754 participants found that two megadoses of vitamin A were effective in reducing mortality from measles in children under two years old and have few associated adverse events. The World Health Organization and UNICEF also recommend Vitamin A to all children diagnosed with measles in areas where mortality is greater than one percent, or where Vitamin A deficiency is a recognized problem.

MENINGOCOCCAL DISEASE

What is it? Meningococcal disease is an acute bacterial infection caused by the bacterium *Neisseria meningitidis*. Symptoms include fever, headache, stiff neck, nausea, vomiting, photophobia, and altered mental status.

Risk of infection: From 2005-2011, there were 0.3 cases of meningococcal disease per one hundred thousand people in the United States.

Overall case-mortality rate: The mortality rate is between ten and fifteen percent.

Treatability: Meningococcal disease can be treated with antibiotics.

MUMPS

What is it? Mumps is an acute viral illness; it spreads through coughing, sneezing, talking, sharing items (such as cups or eating utensils) with others, and touching contaminated objects or surfaces. Symptoms include fever, headache, muscle aches, tiredness, loss of appetite, and swollen and tender salivary glands under the ears on one or both sides. Some people who get mumps have very mild or no symptoms, and often they do not know they have the disease.

Overall case-mortality rate: The mortality rate for mumps is quite small, at less than one percent (0.02 percent, to be exact).

Treatability: There is no cure for mumps; the disease must be allowed to run its course. Treatment focuses on managing symptoms to make the person as comfortable as possible.

PERTUSSIS

What is it? Pertussis (whooping cough) is an acute infectious disease caused by the bacterium *Bordetella pertussis*. The infection is usually spread by coughing or sneezing; you can also contract the illness if you are spending a lot of time and sharing breathing space with an infected person. Early symptoms include runny nose, fever, mild cough, and apnea; after one or two weeks, symptoms include fits of rapid coughing followed by a high-pitched whoop, vomiting during or after coughing fits, and exhaustion after coughing fits.

Risk of infection: Between 1940-1945, there was an average of one hundred and seventy-five thousand cases per year (incidence of approximately one hundred and fifty cases per one hundred thousand people, or 0.15 percent of the population).

Overall case-mortality rate: From 2008 through 2011, a total of seventy-two people died from pertussis; children aged three months or younger accounted for sixty (or eighty-three percent) of these deaths.

Treatability: Pertussis can be treated with antibiotics and with high doses of vitamin C.

PNEUMOCOCCAL INFECTION

What is it? *Streptococcus pneumoniae* causes an acute bacterial infection. The illness spreads from person to person by direct contact with respiratory secretions, like saliva or mucus. Symptoms include fever and chills, cough, rapid breathing, and chest pain.

Risk of infection: There are approximately four hundred thousand hospitalizations from pneumococcal pneumonia annually in the United States (0.1 percent of the population).

Overall case-fatality rate: The case-mortality rate for pneumococcal infection ranges from five to seven percent (higher among the elderly).

Treatability: Pneumococcal disease can be treated with antibiotics.

POLIOMYELITIS

What is it? Poliomyelitis is a viral infection caused by the poliovirus, that affects the nervous system. It enters the body through the mouth and typically spreads through contact with the feces (stool) of an infected person and, less commonly, through droplets from a sneeze or cough.

Most people infected with poliovirus (about seventy-two out of one hundred) will not have any visible symptoms. Twenty-four percent of people will develop a low-grade fever and sore throat, which typically resolves in about one week. Nonparalytic aseptic meningitis occurs in one to five percent of infected individuals. Symptoms of this include stiff neck, back, and legs, followed by symptoms of minor illness lasting two to ten days, then subsequent complete recovery.

Fewer than one percent of all polio infections in children result in flaccid paralysis, and many persons with paralytic poliomyelitis recover completely. From 1980 through 1999, a total of one hundred and sixty-two confirmed cases of paralytic poliomyelitis were reported, an average of eight cases per year.

Overall case-fatality rate: The death-to-case ratio for paralytic polio is generally two to five percent among children and up to between fifteen and thirty percent for adults (depending on age). It increases to between twenty-five and seventy-five percent with bulbar involvement.

Treatability: During a polio outbreak in the late 1940s and early 1950s, Dr. Frederick Klenner, M.D. cured patients of polio with mega-doses of vitamin C. His findings were presented at the annual session of the American Medical Association in 1949.

There are three classifications of paralytic polio:

1. Spinal polio: seventy-nine percent of paralytic cases.

2. Bulbar: two percent of cases.

3. Bulbospinal polio, a combination of bulbar and spinal paralysis: nineteen percent of cases.

ROTAVIRUS

What is it? Rotavirus is a viral gastrointestinal infection found most commonly in infants and young children. Symptoms include severe watery diarrhea, vomiting, fever, abdominal pain, loss of appetite, and dehydration.

Risk of infection: Before the vaccination was introduced, an estimated three million rotavirus infections occurred annually in the United States (one percent of the population).

Overall case-mortality rate: The case-mortality rate for rotavirus is extremely small (0.0001 percent).

Treatability: Treatment for rotavirus focuses on symptom management, mainly drinking plenty of fluids to prevent dehydration.

RUBELLA

What is it? Rubella is a viral infection that is usually mild, especially in children. The virus spreads when an infected person coughs or sneezes. Symptoms include a red rash, fever, headache, mild pink eye, cough, swollen lymph nodes, runny nose, and general discomfort; however, about twenty-five to fifty percent of people infected with rubella will not experience any symptoms.

Risk of infection: The risk of infection with rubella is less than one percent (0.02 percent, to be exact).

Overall case-mortality rate: Rubella can be severe in early gestation and can lead to fetal death, miscarriage, or preterm delivery in pregnant women, but in other populations symptoms are typically mild.

Treatability: Rubella treatment focuses on symptom management until the patient is recovered.

TETANUS

What is it? Tetanus is an acute disease caused by an exotoxin produced by the bacterium *Clostridium tetani*. This illness does not spread from person to person. The bacteria are usually found in soil, dust, and manure and enter the body through breaks in the skin — usually cuts or puncture wounds caused by contaminated objects. Symptoms include jaw cramping, sudden involuntary muscle spasms, painful muscle stiffness, trouble swallowing, seizures, headache, fever, sweating, changes in blood pressure, and rapid heart rate.

Risk of infection: Tetanus is uncommon in the United States, with an average of thirty reported cases each year. From the early 1900s to the late 1940s, there was an estimated 0.4 case per one hundred thousand people; in 2009, there was only 0.1 case per one hundred thousand people.

Overall case-mortality rate: The death-to-case ratio from tetanus has declined from thirty percent to approximately ten percent in recent years.

Treatability: Tetanus is treated with a medicine called human tetanus immune globulin.

VARICELLA

What is it? Varicella (chickenpox) is an acute viral infection caused by the varicella zoster virus (VZV). The illness usually lasts about five to seven days and is typically spread through touching or breathing in the virus particles that come from chickenpox blisters. Infection can also possibly spread through tiny droplets released into the air from infected people when they breathe or talk. Symptoms include a rash that turns into itchy, fluid-filled blisters that eventually turn into scabs; other symptoms include fever, tiredness, loss of appetite, and headache

Risk of complications: Prior to the vaccine, hospitalization rates were approximately two to three per one thousand cases among healthy children.

Overall case-mortality rate: Mortality rates from chickenpox are quite low (0.001 percent).

Treatability: Treatment for varicella focuses on managing symptoms. Calamine lotion and colloidal oatmeal baths may help relieve some of the itching associated with the illness.`

All of the facts are out there; we just aren't always directed to or shown them in their entirety. My advice is to empower yourself to do the research. The time investment into your family's health can pave the road to the greatest reward: a happy, long, and vibrant life.

FOR FURTHER INFORMATION, SEE THE FOLLOWING RESOURCES:

1. Levy, Thomas E. (2002). Vitamin C, Infectious Diseases, and Toxins: Curing the Incurable. Bloomington, IN: Xlibris.
2. Saul, Andrew W. (2007). Hidden in plain sight: The pioneering work of Frederick Robert Klenner, M.D. Journal of Orthomolecular Medicine, 22(1).

3. Huiming, Y, et al. (2005). Vitamin A for treating measles in children. Cochrane Database of Systematic Reviews, 3. https://www.cochranelibrary.com/cdsr/doi/10.1002/14651858.CD001479.pub3/epdf/full

4. Committee on Infectious Diseases. (1993). Vitamin A treatment of measles. Pediatrics, 91(5). https://pediatrics.aappublications.org/content/91/5/1014..info

5. Centers for Disease Control. (2015). The Pink Book: Course Textbook (13th Edition). Atlanta, GA: Centers for Disease Control. Retrieved from www.cdc.gov/vaccines/pubs/pinkbook/index.html.

13

RAISING A CONSCIOUS AND FREE CHILD

By Laira De La Vega

"Thought creates form. This is one of the most powerful concepts that we can teach our children, as this is something that the Machine works very hard to place a hard stop on."

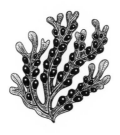

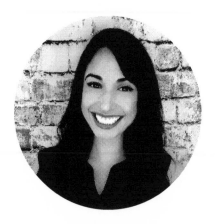

Laira De La Vega is a Certified Reiki Master, trained in NLP and EFT, and is also Director of Vaccine Information for the National Health Federation (NHF.) Laira came into the truth and Human Rights Activism around 2014, shortly after having met her fiance Dr. Russel Myers, who confirmed, in detail, the corrupt truth about vaccines and pharmaceuticals to her, and also the beautiful modalities of chiropractic and natural medicine. Since then, she has worked for many organizations, at different capacities, including having been published in the NHF's Health Freedom News magazine, which circulates globally. After immigrating from Mexico City, MX, as a child, Laira dedicated most of her life to learning about why the World and people are the way they are, and also observed how much Human Rights and freedoms have dissipated over time. During her time as a full time activist, Laira has dedicated herself to fighting for Human Rights and freedoms, and has travelled all over the country to participate in several legislative hearings, full senate hearings, attended the Advisory Committee on Immunization Practices (ACIP), has conducted numerous rallies, been a part of several protests, has educated several lawmakers on the dangers of passing bills that push pharmaceuticals and rob Human Rights, among other areas of activism and advocacy. Laira is now switching gears in helping her community, and will continue to pursue her doctorate in Metaphysics (MhD), as she is fully aware of the turbulent times ahead of this global Awakening, and will help to heal her community, along with other fellow Lightworkers. We are here to serve, in Love & Light.

IN Western societies, most of us grew up in the same world, heavily indoctrinated into a highly controlled "Machine" — the current perceived reality of the world and of how life should be — designed for enslaving its People into obedience. The modern Machine consists of corporate hospitals, the pharmaceutical industry, the public school system, fluoridated water, GMO foods, toxic chemicals in personal care products, TVs, the mainstream media (MSM), the internet, censorship, personal electronic devices, social media, tax-paying corporate America, modern-day expected chronic illness, highly controlled allopathic interventions, and more, all of which have proven to be highly profitable. These are all components of a very well-oiled Machine.

There are a few concepts, or threats, that the Machine strongly disapproves of and has been trying to abolish for quite some time. These threats include:

1. the ability to think and choose freely,
2. the understanding that the "conveniences" offered by the Machine actually take away from us being aware and whole, and
3. the awareness that body and spirit go hand in hand.

The fortunate "problem" here is that many of us have woken up to the fact that not only does this Machine exist but we are the ones who have agreed to its terms and conditions for centuries, even in our ignorance of it. The wonderful news is that there are choices we can make for ourselves and our children that can "unplug" us, and for good.

THE FREE THINKER

Most people believe that freedom simply means the ability to choose things and be able to do them. But there are multiple ways to experience true freedom, including via health, finances, and thought. Part of thinking and choosing freely means having a comprehensive understanding of all facets of reality, including understanding the opposite of freedom, which is what the majority of us have experienced. Seeing the full 360 degree view allows us to make truly informed choices; otherwise we are making choices with incomplete data.

The Machine's typical indoctrination/obedience dynamic begins when we come into this world at birth. Most of us were born in what we thought were the "right" circumstances, with parents obeying the doctor, undergoing an expected, abrasive delivery in a hospital with the mother on her back, bright fluorescent lights blazing, and the current, toxic vaccine schedule in order — thus throwing the newborn baby into the ensnaring grips of the Machine. Some parents realize the truth by looking outside the box to further educate themselves, becoming awakened by friends or family, or finding out the truth the hard way. In this way, some of us, like myself, actually escape the claws of the medical/pharmaceutical indoctrination process and are only partially vaccinated. Others may have been born into families whose parents were fully awake to this corruption and decided against obeying the modern norms; these parents choose to have their children at home, unvaccinated, breastfed, and then raised on real, whole foods. This latter lifestyle is currently frowned upon by the Machine. The forbidden, free-thinking question is: "Why?"

Most of us who are fully awake in the current Machine have always known that something was wrong with the way things were "wired" around us, that something was off about how controlled things are and how obedient so many people have come to be. Some of us were thrown out of classrooms for challenging "authority" regarding what information was being taught, mostly about the accuracy in subjects such as history or religion. The public school system (and the like) has worked very hard to abolish free thinking over time; this is where the obedience perpetuates, going from the paradigm of parents obeying allopathic doctors to children obeying their parents to the child being told to obey authority at school.

Google defines the term "authority" as "the power or right to give orders, make decisions, and enforce obedience." Similarly, the term "obedience" means "compliance with an order, or law or submission to another's authority" and the term "submission" means "the action or fact of accepting or yielding to a superior force or to the will or authority of another person." Think about that. Freely. Think about how these definitions make you feel and the emotions that those words conjure. Then think about this:

"No man is good enough to govern another man without the other's consent" ~ Abraham Lincoln

Are you seeing or feeling a disconnect? If the answer is yes, it is because these statements represent two conflicting dichotomies. One implies obedience and yielding to a superior force, while the other implies freedom.

Authority and obedience are the hallmark of the public school system (and, let's face it, the corporate American workforce), where obedience is instilled, challenging authority is frowned upon, and questioning the taught "facts" is deemed as challenging authority. In that system, our children are not taught how to intend, visualize, meditate, or create or experience abundance and possible ease of life. They are not taught how to live off of the land, nor are they taught about the healing arts of chiropractic or functional medicine. They are not taught how to truly thrive in life. Instead they are taught to simply memorize forced information and to expect and be resigned to a life of hard work, mediocrity, debt, chronic illness, pharmaceutical addiction — ultimately to be an adult worker-bee for and in the well-oiled Machine. Thus this system creates the very programmed, asleep breath of life that helps the profit-making Machine, rather than the people, to thrive.

This is precisely why our children must be taught the "dual truth" — the first truth of what the formerly indoctrinated and now awake individuals have been taught by the Machine and then the rest of the truth that we finally saw after lifting the veil of illusion and waking up to the corruption (very similar to the concept in the movie *The Matrix*). There are several ways in which to inform and empower children gently, without interfering with their innocence. At the end of the day, though, we must teach children what is true rather than what the bulk of society has been led to believe. The fact is that once people start to wake up but are not yet fully disconnected from the Machine, they often fear the process of fully letting go of the old and enslaving way, especially once they get a whiff of true freedom. They have just been taught to obey for so very long. When actually given a license to think and do what they want, many people typically adopt the defense mechanism of becoming very afraid and admitting that they'd rather be told what to do. This is because obedience is all they've ever known. This horrifying mechanism of being afraid of freedom is precisely why we need to equip our children very early on with the proper tools with which to think freely and critically, to recognize and comfortably handle authoritative overreach or abuse, to create healthy boundaries, to respectfully question authority — and all of this before the system programs them with this fearful defense mechanism.

The fact of the matter is that some parents do not have the wherewithal to be able to protect their children in homeschool and ultimately choose to send them into the public school system. Some parents would say that they have no choice at all; that mindset is a direct product of the Machine's indoctrination, as parents have become reliant on the public school system out of the "need" to keep up with modern society. The concept of a healthy work-life balance has now become a thing of the past because the typical Machine-imposed debt and the now normalized forty-hour work week have stolen once normal abilities and freedoms.

However, our children do not belong to the state; they belong to their loving parents, whose responsibilities include teaching them about the importance of many components of free thinking, such as the concept of discernment. This concept is a huge component in thinking and choosing freely; we must be able to receive information without believing it right off the bat. We must do our due diligence and conduct genuine research using credible sources. This goes for everything from the information taught in the public school system to the information received by word of mouth from friends or other people. The latter example is especially important during childhood and adolescence; once in school, children tend to pull away from their families and gravitate toward their peers. Social acceptance becomes central to their self-esteem. This is a very delicate age of awareness in their lives, as these years are a formative time in the building of their adult mindsets. Although children and adolescents tend to want to only listen to what their friends and the media say, we must constantly remind them

to always maintain their sense of individuality and to question everything, no matter how true it might sound.

THE UNPLUGGED CHILD

At today's juncture, kids are born cable-ready and are exposed to
information channels saturated with propagandized misinformation
and disinformation, both of which are ultimately highly profitable to
the Machine. Just as there are components to thinking and choosing
freely, there are also outside influences that need heavy monitoring, as
they tend to keep children "plugged in" very closely to the Machine.
Some of these influences come hidden as information predators. Most
of the mainstream social media platforms that our children and adolescents use are designed with information-mining abilities that leave
our children vulnerable to inadvertently volunteering information. By
design, this helps the Machine get to know them very well. Too well.
Most parents aren't aware of the fact that once they/their kids click "I
agree" to a platform's terms and conditions, they've just allowed the
Machine very intimately into their lives. Information is the Machine's
most precious commodity, as it is basically sheer power. If one of the
Machine's purposes is to abolish free thinking, then it first must know
what thoughts your child is having and what thoughts and decisions
are on the horizon. This process goes beyond childhood and is precisely
why certain government decisions are made — the Machine is always
ten steps ahead. When we volunteer even the slightest information,
even via private message, the Machine gets to know our likes, dislikes,
wants, and needs. We can see examples of this everywhere. All you
have to do is to hop on a social media platform, and you will all of a
sudden say, "Oh wow. I was just talking about that." We must teach our
children the importance of volunteering as little personal information
as possible, not only to prevent the Machine from knowing your child
well but also to prevent any human predator from somehow gaining
access to them.

These external threats work in symphony against the health and
freedom we want for our children, and the Machine perpetuates them

with mental pollution to prevent clear thinking. Electronic entertainment makes up a huge component of this destructive effect. Parents have become too involved in the Machine, with corporate work, debt, and other obligations — so much so that many rely on the convenience of electronic entertainment. This way of life causes major disconnect within personal and family relationships. Not only that — what many people don't know is that by design, these TVs, computers, smartphones, and tablets that we plant in front of our children's faces produce blue light. This blue light can easily damage the retina of the eye, thus potentially causing chronic headaches. Blue light can also disrupt melatonin levels and cause insomnia, which in turn can hinder the body's ability to heal itself. This all places the body in a condition of sympathetic dominance, in a stressed state that can create, intensify, and compound many mental and physical health issues. A body in a stressed state is likely to have raised cortisol levels, which can potentially stop the absorption of nutrients, break down bone and muscle tissue, inhibit proper hormone production, and much more. All of these symptoms typically lead parents to give their children pharmaceuticals in order to mask symptoms that were caused by the Machine itself to begin with. However, free thinking and the type of genuine research that is not taught by or encouraged in the public school system can easily lead parents to this important knowledge.

BODY AND SPIRIT

The reality of true freedom does not just involve choosing to think freely and being cognizant of the physical, destructive components of the Machine; it has so much more to do with a truth that the Machine has worked its hardest to remove from the forefront of our minds. This is the truth that body and spirit go hand in hand. The concept has nothing to do with any religious dogma; rather, it has to do with the components/tools that we are naturally born with, that are part of the construct of the intangible, innate intelligence within and around us. And it all begins with thought.

Thought creates form. This is one of the most powerful concepts that we can teach our children, and it is something that the Machine works very hard to stop. You didn't just look at the palm of your hands and find this book there. An initial thought or idea caused you to somehow have this book in your life. Thought is exactly how this world has unfolded, been shaped, and technically advanced. What the Machine has done is provide its conveniences and quick fixes, in the form of electronic devices, food-like products, and pills, in order to suppress thoughts that can potentially shape the future and create better form. Everyone is born into different circumstances and lives their lives "playing the cards they were dealt." People don't understand that all that can change and that there is great power behind thought and intention. By living our lives as they are, never intending or asking life for anything different, we are just asking life for more of the same. People forget that we are energy and that life responds to the vibration we give off by reflecting back to us the very same. This is why miserable people who are in a constant state of stress continue to attract more of the same; all they do is complain. Joyful people, on the other hand, tend to remain in a state of gratitude. Actually making the choice to have a different attitude can change our entire lives. We alone are accountable for our lives and how it all unfolds. This is a great aspect to experiencing freedom.

Utilizing thought and intention properly can be very successful, especially when combined with silencing the mind. Silence helps us process what is going on around us in the world. People no longer sit still and reflect, nor do they go outside and connect with nature, which has also proven to improve mental/physical health. Such actions are now seen as boring; this is because the information-mining, via electronic devices and such, is always in our faces, feeding us and our children with misinformation and propaganda, distracting us from the beautiful world outside of the Machine. These conveniences suppress our naturally flowing thought, thus preventing us from shaping the future as we would really want it. Human thoughts, ideas, and intentions have literally shaped this entire world throughout time. However, now people are always in a state of confusion or at a loss for what they really want or should do. If we allow the mind some silence, we could find out what it is that we really want, or perhaps an original idea could surface that we had not thought of before. We could potentially be inspired or discover solutions rather than have the Machine's device show us or tell us "our only options."

A very easy and scientifically proven way to naturally silence the mind, provide mental clarity, and lower cortisol levels is through meditation. Meditation doesn't have to mean praying with monks in Tibet. It can be as simple as sitting in nature or in the comfort of your own home, closing your eyes, and focusing on your breath for at least ten to fifteen minutes. Initially, both adults and children will experience some mind chatter; however, if you just let the chatter dissolve without force and come back to focusing on your breathing, it will eventually become very easy. In meditation, people can have less stress, more mental clarity, and elevated moods; they can also find sought-for answers and great wisdom within themselves. If children learn to incorporate meditation as a routine in their lives, you will see an exceptional difference between them and those solidly plugged into the machine. You might have yourself a healthier and more free thinker.

Another direct result of regular meditation is heightened intuition; gut instincts/hunches become more and more accurate with your new mental, physiological, and spiritual clarity. This is very important for you and your child to pay close attention to. Recall the conflicting dichotomies mentioned under "The Free Thinker," how one implied obedience and yielding to a superior force and the other implied freedom. I suggested that you think about how that makes you feel and the emotions that those words conjure. If you felt not-good feelings in association with obedience and submission, this is because those concepts are inherently wrong. If you felt good feelings in relation to the concept of freedom, this is because that freedom is inherently good. These distinctions will become clearer and clearer, and your sharpened emotional compass will greatly assist in providing extra guidance to you and your child throughout life.

My best advice to you is to always talk to your children, especially about how they are feeling. Listen to them, encourage them to ask questions, equip them with the tools that the Machine will never provide. This education in creating freedom is invaluable to both you and your child, and you must start at home in leading by example. Implement these actions alongside your child so that it will be a norm to bring clarity and health into their lives:

1. Think freely.
2. Ask questions/research.
3. Disconnect yourselves from electronic devices.
4. Go outside to connect with nature and meditate.
5. Know that we are energy and that life responds to the vibration we give off by reflecting back to us the very same.
6. Listen to yourself and your child.
7. Intend for new things, and give thanks to life in advance . . .

. . . because you and your child will now be aware and, most importantly, free.

14

NUTRITION AND HEALTHY CHILDREN

By Julie A. Miller, B.S.; A.C.N.

"Don't let food become a power struggle, mealtime should be fun and enjoyable for the entire family."

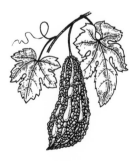

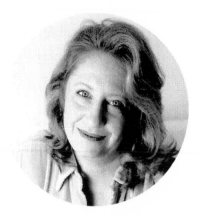

Julie Miller is an applied clinical nutritionist (ACN) in Southern California. A sought-after source for health and functional nutrition information, she has spoken to large corporations and community groups and has been a resource for wellness programs.

Julie practices nutrition as part of Miller Family Health. The practice has been established for over thirty-five years; as a result, they have multi-generation families as patients. She has also developed a close relationship with the local midwifery community in her area and has a large family-oriented practice.

Julie's journey to nutrition was indirect. She spent years in corporate management and accounting but was not satisfied. After she lost both her parents at early ages to different diseases, health and nutrition became a high priority for Julie. While she was raising her young family, she always had some natural healing or nutrition book close by in order to look up remedies. When it came time to reinvent herself with a new career, it was not surprising that nutrition became Julie's next venture.

Julie's patients know that she will go to extreme lengths to facilitate their healing, from experimenting in the kitchen to revise a patient's favorite recipe into a "healthy version" without losing the flavor and teaching cooking classes to demonstrating exercises, stretches, and yoga poses and teaching breathing exercises. Julie will do whatever is required to take care of the whole person.

www.millerfamilycare.com/julie-miller/
fb: @MillerFamilyCare

We are making so many technological advances in healthcare, yet as a population, we are becoming sicker. There are now over one hundred and fifty different autoimmune diseases, and we now recognize diseases never previously associated with children as Contemporary Chronic Childhood illnesses. We try to outsmart diseases and have adopted the attitude that we should avoid illness and disease at all costs. However, the immune system was designed to be challenged in order to develop and strengthen. By taking all "childhood disease" away, we are taking away the training ground for the immune system to develop and learn naturally.

As omnivores, we have many choices about the food we eat. Furthermore, in our modern society, we do not have to forage or raise all of our food. We have the convenience of grocery stores, specialty markets, delivery services, restaurants, food prep services, and more at our disposal. Gone are the restrictions that dictated what we could gather or grow seasonally. We now have access to tropical fruits or tomatoes, as well as to lots of other options, all year round. The problem with this easy availability of food is that the consumers are far removed from the process.[218]

As a nutritionist, my philosophy is to meet the patient where they are and guide them to make small changes toward a healthier lifestyle. My father-in-law, Milton Miller, D.C., was a great healer who taught me many things. One of his favorite sayings was, "Someone convinced against their will is of the same opinion still." In other words, I am not able to change another person's beliefs by butting heads with them; however, I may be able to convince them to accept small changes a little at a time.

Whether you would like to live a vegan, paleo, keto, or Mediterranean lifestyle, there may be room for dietary improvement to achieve your goals. I have met vegetarians who do not eat many vegetables but consume large amounts of grains; similarly, I've met people pursuing a keto lifestyle for specific health reasons yet consuming large quantities of processed meats. Wherever we are on our health journey, we all have room for improvement as long as we are open to accepting some guidance.

INTRODUCING FIRST FOODS

Businesses face pressure to continually improve their financial performance, which can only happen if they increase revenue while cutting their expenses. Agriculture is no different. Producers and processors face pressure to turn a crop faster, fatten and sell the stock sooner, use cheaper materials, cut corners. To combat these shortfalls in food quality, we can begin by presenting our children with real food.

Historically, we have introduced cereal as a first food after breast milk or formula at approximately four to six months of age. The rationale is that something heavier will help babies sleep through the night and not be as hungry. However, the body needs enzymes in order to digest the starchy carbohydrates found in cereal. Amylase (an enzyme that aids in digestion) is needed to break down starches; babies do not make enough of this enzyme to handle a starchy food like cereal, even when it is mixed with breast milk. A human first produces amylase between six months to two years of age, but the development of enough amylase in the digestive process usually coincides with the development of molars. In other words, even if your baby begins amylase production at six months, they will not be capable of handling starches yet at that age. Too early an introduction to simple starches like cereal can lead to digestive complications and/or allergies, both of which affect babies' gut function and ultimately immune systems. This can set the stage for their overall health for life.

So what are the best foods to begin with? Since simple carbohydrates are off the table, better to start with fats and proteins.

Think of how much babies grow and develop during their first year of life. At first, they are bundles of cuteness, completely reliant on others for all of their needs. They require fats to support brain development and the body's communication system: the nervous system.

In addition, the amino acids in protein provide the essential building blocks for healthy tissues, muscles, and organs.

For babies approximately six months old, ideal foods to start with include egg yolks, bone broths, liver, and other pureed proteins. Additionally, avocado and coconut oil, which contain good fats, and banana, which has amylase (the enzyme that breaks down carbohydrates), are good places to begin. Once a baby can tolerate bananas, we can add cooked and strained apricots, apples, and pears to the diet. If the consistency of the puree is too thick, you can thin it with a little pure water or breast milk.

FOOD FOR BABIES AND TODDLERS

We are all unique . . . children, cultures, families. We all have our preferences, our likes and dislikes. The most important thing to remember with toddlers is NOT to make food a battleground. Children have very little control over their environment. With food, however, they have a say in what they will or will not eat. Sometimes it can become a tug-of-war or a game of wills.

The best option for introducing new foods to toddlers is to set the expectation that one day, they may be ready for a different taste or food. Place a tiny amount of the new food on their plate and say something like, "Just see if you are old enough to like this yet." If they don't like it, just leave it or take it away and thank them for trying. By about the fifth time we introduce a food, it is no longer "foreign" and may be accepted; however, in some cases it can take up to fifteen exposures for a child to accept a new food. Don't give up too soon. It is important to introduce and expose children to foods, smells, and experiences for a rich environment and to set the stage for lifelong learning.

COMMONLY SUGGESTED FOODS TO AVOID

Cold breakfast cereal is often used as a packageable snack for toddlers. It is easy to transport and hand to the kids in the car and easy for them to hold and manipulate. I get the simplicity. Life can be challenging, and we are all looking for those things that make it just a little bit easier.

Using cereal as an example, though, let me make the argument for "real" food — food that has not been through loads of processes and/or chemically altered. Let's begin with what cereals contain: a lot of GMOs. We even find GMOs in the brands we think to be healthier.[219] Beware the label "natural"; it does not always mean as clean as we think.[220]

Next, we contend with the word "fortified." When a product is fortified, it means that the company has added back in synthetic vitamins and minerals. I will use vitamin C as an example. The chemical formula for ascorbic acid is $C_6H_8O_6$. The medical community often considers this compound to be vitamin C; however, real vitamin C in its natural form contains enzymes and co-enzymes that aid in making the vitamin bioavailable and usable to the body. Whole vitamin C also contains phytonutrients and bio-flavonoids, which provide antioxidant and anti-inflammatory activities. Tyrosinase, an enzyme that aids in the regulation of the production of melanin, also comprises a piece of vitamin C. There are also P, K, and J factors. The P factors help strengthen blood vessels; think bloody nose and bruising. The K factors are necessary for blood clotting.[221] The J factor aids the process of oxygen binding with red blood cells. Vitamin C-rich foods are plentiful in nature. They include broccoli, Brussels sprouts, bell peppers, spinach, squash, tomatoes, sweet potatoes, kiwi, berries, and more. However, in our modern food production system, the majority of ascorbic acid is derived from corn sugar, which is almost always derived from GMO corn (of which there is an abundance). Corn sugar is not a healthy sugar for anyone to include in their diet.

The process of making cold cereal presents another real problem. The process is called extrusion; it uses high temperatures and pressure, which destroys a lot of the nutrients, particularly proteins, in the ingredients being processed. The severe process changes the structure of proteins, rendering the end product toxic to the nervous system.[222]

SUPPORTING A HEALTHY IMMUNE SYSTEM

Nutritionally, many micronutrients support the immune system. By exposing children to a variety of foods, including ample fruits and vegetables, we can ensure that they are getting the necessary vitamins and minerals to stay healthy. Consuming an actual rainbow of food is the immune system's best defense against infection and viruses. Foods such as carrots, plums, apricots, sweet potatoes, kale, spinach, cantaloupe, squash, tomatoes, grapes, berries, broccoli, apples, spinach, and chard (to name just a few) are rich in micronutrients.

WHAT IS SO GREAT ABOUT BONE BROTH?

Since man discovered fire, we have been making soup. Every culture on Earth has at least one soup recipe. From Viet Nam, we get pho; we get rasam from India, egg drop from China, borscht from the Ukraine, miso from Japan, and lentil with spinach from Ethiopia. The reason is simple: soup is a great way to pack a lot of nutrition into a meal.

The resurgence of bone broth can most likely be attributed to the paleo movement. We can get some great things from bone broth to help keep us healthy.[223] Bone broth is the best nutritional source of collagen, which is important for building healthy connective tissue, ligaments, tendons, skin, muscles, and bones. Collagen also relates to a healthy immune system because the same cells that make up our skin also line our digestive tract. These cells are designed to connect tightly together so we can take baths and showers without absorbing all the water and so that we keep our insides where they belong. Having a healthy digestive tract improves our immunity because approximately seventy percent of our innate immune function stems from our gut health. A healthy digestive lining means a happier gut environment.

BONE BROTH WITH ROASTED GARLIC

WHAT YOU NEED:

- 4 pounds beef bones
- 1/2 bunch celery, coarsely chopped
- 1 onion, coarsely chopped
- 4 medium carrots, scrubbed and coarsely chopped
- 1 tablespoon tomato paste **or** 1T apple cider vinegar **or** 1T lemon juice
- 3T olive oil
- 1 head garlic, halved crosswise
- 1 bunch herbs, including stems (parsley, cilantro, thyme, rosemary)
- 4 bay leaves
- 1/2 teaspoon black peppercorns
- 1/2 teaspoon coriander seeds

INSTRUCTIONS:

1. Line a baking sheet with parchment paper. Preheat oven to four hundred and fifty degrees Fahrenheit. Place bones on prepared baking sheet and vegetables on prepared pan and roast twenty minutes. Spread the tomato paste over the bones and vegetables and roast for an additional five minutes; set aside.

2. Transfer the bones and vegetables to a slow cooker and cover with cold water; if you did not use tomato paste, add apple cider vinegar or lemon juice. Add the herbs, bay leaves, peppercorns, and coriander seeds. Set on low and let cook for eight to ten hours. Strain and discard solids.

* Can freeze for up to three months.

* Mix ratios to preferred consistency; do not use a metal spoon or container, as the metal will leach into the mixture.

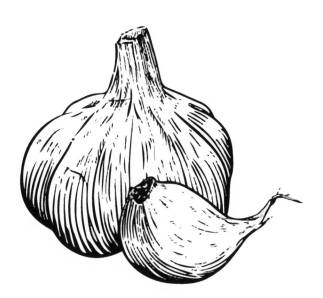

OMEGA 3 SUPPLEMENT

If you Google omega 3's and children, you'll get 122,000,000 results in .61 seconds. It has been long understood that fat is important for brain health and development. Adequate amounts of omega 3s are needed for the brain, vision, and proper neurotransmitter metabolism.[224]

Cod liver oil is one of those things that was in fashion for a very long time, went out of fashion for a while, and is back. In addition to omega 3, cod liver oil is also a natural source of vitamins A and D. The list of omega 3's benefits is long. It supports brain development; it is anti-inflammatory; it provides nourishment for hair, skin, and nails; it supports healthy bones and vision; it strengthens the heart and helps overall immunity. While someone who is very healthy and has a well-founded diet has little need to take supplements, I make an exception for a good omega 3 supplement because our diets tend to lack adequate amounts of this crucial fat. I recommend finding as clean a source as possible, as well as one that is cold pressed to preserve its nutritional value. If you are vegan, you could consider a source from seaweed or algae. Cod liver oil can be given to babies as young as three months; use a few drops and gradually adjust the dose as they age until they receive an adult dose at twelve years old.

THE ROLE OF SLEEP

Food is important to our health but so is getting enough sleep. When we sleep, the body experiences repair and growth. A newborn sleeps an average of sixteen to eighteen hours a day. That sleep is necessary for proper development and growth to occur. Too little sleep can suppress immune function. If the immune system is not at its optimal level, it cannot fight colds and flus.[225][226]

THE ROLE OF EXERCISE

Exercise is crucial for both physical and mental health, but the role of exercise in children's health is often overlooked. We have lots of distractions vying for our attention, and children are not exempt: television, computer games, phones, and apps. It is important to make time to incorporate daily exercise in our children's lives.

Exercise produces endorphins, the "feel good" hormone, which result in happier children. It is also a good way to work off some energy so that when it comes time to sit, study, or sleep, the mind is much calmer. Children who regularly engage in exercise see a marked decrease of reported depression.[227] Exercise influences positive outcomes for mood and behavior in two ways. First, it concentrates activity in areas of the brain responsible for coordination, agility, and focus instead of in areas of the brain that deal with worry, frustration, anxiety, fear, and anger. Second, aerobic exercise influences actual brain chemistry, particularly when it comes to the support of neurotransmitters that control behavior or impulse control.

Regular exercise in children also produces strong bones and muscles.[228] In addition, children who exercise on average have higher self-esteem, coordination, posture, and balance. Exercise develops a strong heart and builds endurance. In terms of immune function, exercise is thought to flush out bacteria and reduce the chances of getting a cold or flu; it also has a positive effect on immune-fighting white blood cells and the upregulation of antibodies. The increase in body temperature caused by exercise aids in fighting infection. Finally, exercise ultimately acts as an aid in stress reduction; some evidence shows that exercise reduces the production of stress hormones.[229] To get children to incorporate exercise into their daily lives, we can encourage lots of fun activities, including dance, martial arts, tennis, skating, soccer, and swimming, to name just a few.

Keeping both the mind and the body strong with nutrition, sleep, and exercise will build a foundation for a lifetime of better health and immune function.

15

FROM THE FARMACY

By Lesa Ritchie Craig, HHC

"The gut is the gateway to a strong immune system."

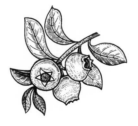

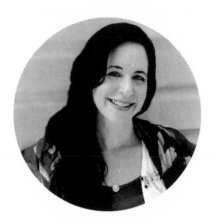

Lesa Craig is a holistic health coach and a self-proclaimed nutrition nerd with a passion for mind, body, and gut balance. As a wife of a retired Army veteran and mother of seven, she defines her family as the "why" that inspires her to take on every challenge with a positive attitude. In 2008, she dramatically changed her family's diet after she and her children experienced a series of health issues: Autism Spectrum Disorder, failure to thrive, seizures, severe allergies, heavy metal overload, systemic yeast, constipation, ADHD, anxiety disorder, asthma, autoimmune disorders, and developmental delays. It has been no small undertaking. While battling her own addiction to sugar, she decided to take matters into her own hands and enrolled in The Institute for Integrative Nutrition. She graduated from IIN in 2011, received her drugless practitioner license, and continues to study leading nutrition science. She and her husband run Vibrant Families Health and Wellness, empowering others to take control of their own health.

www.vibrantfamilies.com

You need not know everything about macrophages, T cells, and B cells to understand that your complex immune system is affected by what you put in your body. Viruses, bacteria, fungi, and protozoa pathogens are everywhere, and our immune system is our first line of defense in protecting us from these invaders.[230] But the toxins in our food, our environment, and our vaccines play a direct role in depleting our immune system. Most everyone today has toxic overload, which manifests in each individual body in various ways. How can you keep your children, and yourself, healthy in a toxic world? Building a strong immune system begins in the gut.[231][232] Approximately eighty percent of our entire immune system is in the gut wall.[233] Good nutrition can support the immune response and help eliminate toxic overload in the body; however, our bodies must be able to digest food before we can absorb necessary nutrients efficiently.

When my son was seven years old, he was diagnosed with ASD (Autism Spectrum Disorder). We started with a gluten-free and casein-free diet. However, after allergy testing, we discovered he was allergic to not only wheat and dairy but also all the foods we had replaced them with. He was literally allergic to everything but cockroach and mouse urine. I felt completely lost and overwhelmed about how to help my child. We focused on healing his digestive tract and improving his microbiome using bone broth and L-Glutamine. We created a food journal and continued to expand the number of superfoods we could eat. Now, ten years later, that same child can eat almost anything, and he loves to cook.

You may not have control over every pathogen you or your child come into contact with, but you can decide what you put on your plates. I encourage everyone to allow kids to be part of the journey, create and explore recipes together, and challenge their taste buds. Praise your child for trying something new. Celebrate your health and have *fun* with food. There are endless recipes using superfoods to boost and strengthen your immune system. In this chapter, I will share a few of my family's favorites, along with some tips for the pickiest eaters.

"Let food be thy medicine and medicine be thy food" ~Hippocrates

TEN QUICK TIPS FOR HEALTHY EATING

1. Let kids help in the kitchen.

2. Eat more vegetables, especially leafy greens. Make eating greens fun!

3. Eat a rainbow of fruits and vegetables. Do a daily rainbow challenge with your kids.

4. Eat whole foods, organic when possible. Eliminate complex carbs like breads and pasta.

5. Eat fermented foods: kefir, kombucha, kimchi, sauerkraut, and miso.

6. Turn kids into food detectives. Teach them how read the packages. Read ingredients before nutrition facts. If you can't pronounce it, don't eat it!

7. Eat nutrient-loaded foods. Count quality over quantity; calories are not created equal.

8. No GMOs or artificial ingredients. No artificial sugars, preservatives, or colors.

9. Avoid added sugar. If you add sugar to a recipe, try dates, honey, real maple syrup, or organic raw sugar, but always in moderation. A safe no-calorie sweetener is Molokai fruit.

10. Drink more water.

IMMUNE-BOOSTING SUPERFOODS

- Leafy greens, kale, and broccoli
- Berries
- Onions and garlic
- Turmeric
- Mushrooms
- Beans and legumes
- Bone broths
- Cacao
- Ginger
- Fermented foods
- Avocado
- Nuts and seeds

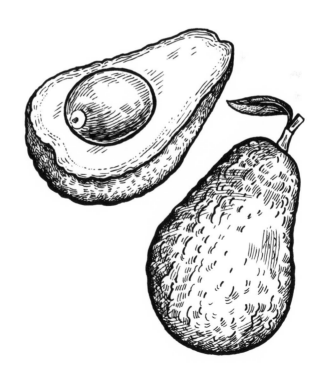

"MORE KALE PLEASE!" KALE SALAD

8-12 servings

I often hear my kids say, "I love kale!" or "More kale, please!" Kale is an anti-inflammatory, antioxidant, and anticarcinogen and is also a prebiotic, supporting your microbiome and immune system.[234] It is also rich in vitamins C, A, and K, iron, folate and calcium.[235] Kids love to help make this salad because they get to work with their hands and choose the ingredients. Allowing kids to help and make choices encourages them to eat healthier foods. They feel proud of their creations and they learn about the power of each superfood. The trick to making kale salad taste amazing is massaging the leaves, which little helping hands do well. Secret ingredients: love and fun!

WHAT YOU NEED:

- 2 head of curly kale
- 1/3 cup of liquid aminos or soy sauce
- 2 Tbsp. fresh squeezed calamansi, limes, or lemons
- 1 pinch of sea salt
- 1/2 cup of olive oil
- 1 cup of green onion, diced
- 1/2 medium red onion, diced
- 2 cloves of garlic, minced
- 1 cup halved cherry tomatoes
- 1/2 jicama, cut into slivers
- 1 cup variety of colorful peppers
- 1 carrot, shredded
- 1 avocado, cubed
- Add any of your favorite fruits, vegetables, or cooked quinoa
- Handful of seeds: pepitas/pumpkin seeds, sesame seeds, sunflower seeds, hemp seeds

INSTRUCTIONS:

1. Remove the leaves of the kale from the stalks. Tear the kale into bite-sized pieces and place in a large bowl.
2. Add the liquid aminos/soy sauce, fresh-squeezed juice, sea salt, and olive oil. Massage the ingredients into the kale leaves. This helps break down the leaves so they are no longer bitter. Work your leaves for about five minutes, ensuring that no leaf is left unturned.
3. Add additional vegetables and toss. This is where you can get creative with this recipe and really make it your own. Add vegetables and fruits you love. I aim for color and taste: purple carrots, red, orange, and yellow peppers, and even blueberries and pineapple.
4. Marinate in the fridge for about three hours. Add any nuts and seeds just before serving. Kale salad can last in the fridge for about a week, if it doesn't disappear before then!

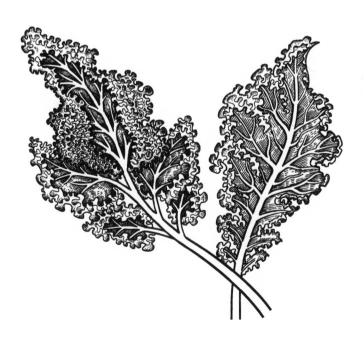

KALE CHIPS

About 6-8 servings

Kale chips are another kale favorite in my house, especially with my four-year-old. They are so easy and quick. We can pop these in the oven, and they make a great crunchy snack — helpful as appetizers for hungry kids. My four-year-old can finish a whole batch by himself!

WHAT YOU NEED:

- 1 bunch of curly kale
- 1 Tbsp olive oil
- 1 tsp sea salt or other seasoning to taste

INSTRUCTIONS:

1. Be sure to wash and dry kale in advance so the leaves are not soggy. Tear kale into bite-sized pieces and add them to a large bowl.
2. Add olive oil and seasoning and coat the leaves lightly.
3. Spread the kale pieces out on a parchment-lined baking sheet. Sprinkle any additional seasoning per your preference.
4. Bake at three hundred degrees Fahrenheit for eight to twelve minutes, or until the kale is crisp and just before the edges start to brown. Watch the end process closely; they can become over-cooked quickly.

CHOCOLATE AVOCADO CHIA SEED PUDDING

Serves 6-8

My kids simply refer to this as chocolate pudding, but it is packed so full of nutrients that it could almost be a meal rather than a dessert. Raw cacao has one of the highest levels of antioxidants of any superfood. It is also rich in magnesium, calcium, and iron and is a natural antidepressant.[236] Chia seeds are packed with protein, fiber, and calcium and are high in omega 3's.[237] Avocados surprisingly pair nicely with chocolate; these little green fruits really make this pudding so smooth and creamy. Avocados also contain powerful amounts of vitamins, including vitamin K and folate, as well as more potassium than bananas.[238] Their healthy fats are also beneficial for helping your body absorb nutrients.

WHAT YOU NEED:

- 3-4 avocados
- 3/4 cup raw cacao powder
- 2 Tbsp chia seeds
- 2 Tbsp coconut cream
- 3/4 cup coconut milk
- 1 tsp vanilla extract (optional)
- Pinch of sea salt
- 3/4 cup honey or other sweetener of choice

INSTRUCTIONS:

1. Combine all ingredients into the blender and blend until smooth. Add additional coconut milk for desired thickness.
2. Divide into individual serving dishes and chill for at least an hour.

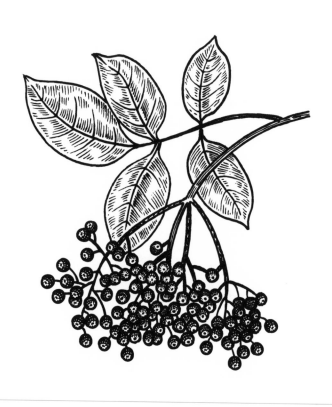

BLACK ELDERBERRY SYRUP

Makes 2-3 cups

Elderberries (Sambucus) have been an ancient medicine for centuries. Elderberries work as a powerful antiviral, antibacterial, antimicrobial, anti-inflammatory, and antioxidant. Elderberry extract and syrup can provide a significant boost to the immune system, both as a preventative and as a treatment.[239] Studies show a reduction of cold and flu duration and severity, with individuals recovering one to four days faster with elderberry treatment.[240] Making your own elderberry syrup is so easy and can save you money compared to store-bought brands. The best part is you know exactly what is in it and can tweak it to be your own.

WHAT YOU NEED:

- 1 cup dried organic elderberries (100g)*
- 6 cups of cold filtered water
- 1 cup sweetener: raw honey** or maple syrup, coconut sugar, monk fruit

Optional variations:
- 1 tsp cinnamon or 1 cinnamon stick (add to the boil)
- 1/2 tsp ground cloves (add to the boil)
- 2-3 tsp of ground ginger (add to the boil)
- 1 drop wild orange essential oil (add once cooled)
- 2 Tbsp apple cider vinegar (add once cooled)

*Do NOT eat elderberries raw.

**Never feed honey to babies under a year old; if using honey, allow your syrup to cool to preserve the quality of the honey.

INSTRUCTIONS:

1. Place berries in cold water in a large saucepan and allow them to soak for about an hour until they are soft.
2. Add optional cinnamon, cloves, and/or ginger. Place over medium heat and gradually bring to a rolling boil.
3. Reduce to simmer and cook another forty-five minutes, stirring frequently. Do not cover the pot.
4. Remove from heat and let steep for one hour.
5. Strain the berries and liquid through a fine mesh strainer or use a cheesecloth and squeeze out the liquid. If you are adding essential oils and apple cider vinegar, you can add it in this step. You should have two cups of liquid when done; add filtered water if you don't have two cups. Stir until well combined.
6. Transfer the syrup to a sterilized glass jar and store in the fridge. You can keep this up to two weeks in the fridge; you can also store in the freezer. Freeze the syrup in ice cube trays for individual servings. You could also make elderberry popsicles (*see Vitamin C popsicles*).

Prevention dosage for children sone year and older:

20-30 lbs: ½ tsp twice a day

30-90 lbs: 1 tsp twice a day

Adults: 1-2 tsp twice a day

Treatment dosage for children one year and older:

20-30 lbs: ½ tsp every 4 hours

30-90 lbs: 1 tsp every 4 hours

Adults: 1-2 tsp every 4 hours

VITAMIN C POPSICLES

Makes 16 popsicles in ½ cup molds

These popsicles will boost vitamin C, which works as a prevention and a treatment when kids are sick. They will also keep kids happy and hydrated. I follow Dr. Suzanne Humphries' vitamin C protocol, using a powder crystalline form of ascorbic acid.[241] You can add elderberry syrup for an extra immune boost, or you can add greens or additional supplements. My children can easily go through three or four popsicles a day when they are sick.

WHAT YOU NEED:

- 2 cups of frozen mangoes
- 1 cup of frozen pineapple
- 1 QT coconut water
- Additional filtered water
- 4 tsp of powdered vitamin C/ascorbic acid (1600mg)
- 2 Tbsp raw honey

Optional:
- Elderberry syrup
- Echinacea
- Cinnamon
- Substitute any frozen fruit
- Add fresh or powdered greens for added nutrients
- Alternative sweeteners

INSTRUCTIONS:

1. Place all ingredients in a blender; blend until smooth.
2. Add enough water to equal eight cups, and blend again to mix thoroughly.
3. Add to individual popsicle molds and freeze.

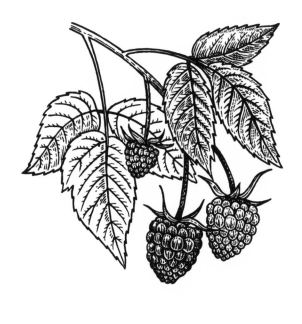

VERY BERRY SMOOTHIE

Serves 4-6

Berry smoothies are the best way to hide greens from picky eaters because the berries are so bright that you can't see green. My oldest son used to say he was allergic to green when he was little; now broccoli is his favorite. The trick with adding greens is to start slowly, and eventually the taste buds will crave them. For this recipe, I use a total of only a half cup of greens. You can start with even less for super picky kids. Powdered greens that have a variety of vegetables and fruit are also a good option. This may be the only way to get some kids to eat greens in the beginning. I add protein to this smoothie as well so it becomes a complete meal — real "fast food" that you can take on the go!

WHAT YOU NEED:

- 3 cups frozen mixed berries
- 1/2 cup of ice
- 1/4 cup spinach
- 1/4 cup kale (remove stem or use baby kale)
- 2 cups coconut milk
- Additional water

Optional
- 1Tbps flax, chia, and/or hemp seeds
- 1 scoop protein powder
- 1 scoop mixed greens powder
- 1/2 tsp turmeric
- 2 Tbsp raw honey

INSTRUCTIONS:

1. Place all ingredients in a blender and blend until smooth.
2. Add water until you reach your ideal consistency. Enjoy!

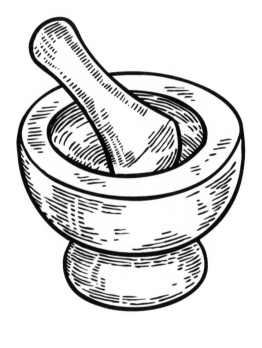

THE ULTIMATE FLU-SHOT

6-8 Servings

We make this during "cold and flu" season or during high travel times. This recipe is meant to be 2-4oz shots, not a full smoothie. You can cut this recipe in half, but I usually make a batch for the whole family at once. Then I yell for the kids, "Come get your flu-shot!" When people ask if we got our flu shot this year, I respond with, "Yes, several times. We make it ourselves, and it tastes great!"

WHAT YOU NEED:

- 2 cups frozen mangoes
- 2 Tbsp elderberry syrup
- 2 droppers super echinacea
- 2 tsp vitamin C
- 1/2 tsp chlorella
- 10-20 drops of liquid D-3 *depending on the dose and number of servings
- 1 Tbsp of raw honey (optional)
- 4 cups coconut water

INSTRUCTIONS:

1. Place all ingredients in the blender and blend until smooth. Enjoy!

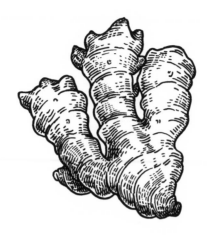

NATURAL ANTIBIOTIC ELIXIR

6-8 Servings

My family deals with two major issues when it comes to prescription antibiotics. We have allergies to sulfa and penicillin, and we already deal with gut imbalance. Prescription antibiotics kill all bacteria, both the good and the bad. In addition, prescription antibiotics are only good for bacterial infection and won't touch viral or fungal infections. I created this elixir because it is an amazing and powerful antibiotic, as well as an antiviral and antifungal. It will not deplete the friendly bacteria; instead, it actually supports the overall immune health. This concoction will fight even the strongest super drug-resistant bacteria, like MRSA, as well as viruses.[242, 243, 244, 245]

You can make this elixir as potent as you feel necessary. A secret tip to getting kids to take an elixir or any adverse flavor is to numb the tongue. You can do this by letting them eat part of a vitamin C Popsicle or sucking on an ice cube first. Then use a medicine dispenser/oral syringe and squirt the elixir way in the back of the mouth. Afterward, give them a spoonful of raw or Manuka honey or the rest of their Popsicle to hide the flavor.

WHAT YOU NEED:

- 4 fresh garlic cloves, peeled and crushed
- 1" fresh ginger, grated
- 1/4 tsp turmeric, ground or freshly grated
- 1/2 cup raw or Manuka honey
- 2 Tbsp raw organic apple cider vinegar
- 2 lemons, squeezed (about 1/2 cup)
- 1/2 cup filtered water
- 1/4 tsp organic cinnamon (or 1 drop of essential oil)
- 1 dash of cayenne

INSTRUCTIONS:

1. Place all ingredients in a blender and blend until smooth.
2. Take 1/2 tsp-1 tsp every two hours at the height of the illness and then once or twice a day as needed until recovery. This will last about five days in the fridge. The garlic will be most beneficial just after being freshly chopped, so you may want to add freshly chopped garlic daily.

WHAT'S IN THE MEDICINE CABINET?

You should have naturopathic and homeopathic remedies available to use when the first signs of infection or illness appear. You can handle most illnesses at home, but always seek the advice of a licensed practitioner if you are unsure. Support the body's natural ability to fight off any foreign pathogens and return to a calm, healthy normal. Show gratitude for your body and nourish it with superfoods and love. Support the process. Trust your instincts.

Cannabidiol (CBD) oil: CBD oil creates balance and homeostasis throughout the immune and central nervous systems. Know your source for CBD oil — it should be non-GMO and pesticide-free, as well as third-party tested to contain therapeutic levels of CBD.[246, 247]

Epsom salts: Epsom salts contain magnesium, which helps rid the body of toxins and reduce inflammation. An Epsom salt bath promotes relaxation and reduces stress, pain, and swelling.

Essential oils: Always use a good quality brand like DoTerra or Young Living. You should also know which oils are kid-safe. I always have lavender, frankincense, helichrysum, lemon, lime, cinnamon, Roman chamomile, peppermint, and melaleuca. My favorite DoTerra blends are OnGuard, Breathe, and Brave. DoTerra also sells kids-only blends in a roller so they are so easy to use.

Homeopathic: I like Hyland's and Boiron. These companies both sell a first aid homeopathic kits and kids' kits and also explain how to use them. The ones I keep on hand are calendula (cream and pellets), arnica (ointment, cream, and pellets), Cold Calm, Oscillococcinum, belladonna, chamomilla, and thuja.

Vitamin C: Already mentioned but worth mentioning again: Dr. Suzanne Humphries recommends sodium ascorbate, crystalline. Make sure your source is reputable and non-GMO. It should be just vitamin C; avoid complex vitamins when trying to take high doses because you'll end up taking too much of the additional ingredients. Dr. Humphries recommends Nutribiotic brand, Liposomal Sodium Ascorbate, and Livon Labs.

Vitamin D-3 ("The Sunshine Vitamin"): If you are getting enough outdoor sunshine (fifteen minutes a day without sunscreen or long sleeves), you may not need a supplement. But during the fall and winter, our vitamin D levels drop. My favorite brands of vitamin D are Metagenics, Carlson, and Nordic Naturals. Always choose a reputable company and research where they source their ingredients.

Echinacea: I prefer super echinacea tincture, which uses the whole organic plant, including the leaf, stem, flower, and seed. My kids will take this straight. You can purchase an alcohol-free version.

Chlorella: Chlorella is an amazing detoxifier and supports your immune system. This will help get the heavy metals and other toxins out of the body while enhancing B-vitamin and protein intake.

Protein powder and powdered greens: Keep a good quality protein powder and powdered version of super greens on hand to turn smoothies into a quick, complete meal. Do your research and choose a product from a reputable source with high-quality ingredients. Ensure that there are no artificial ingredients, especially artificial sugars.

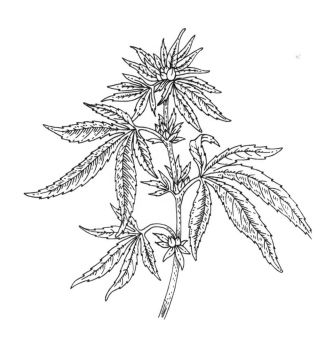

Endnotes

1   Trimble, Megan. (2018, January 11). U.S. kids more likely to die than kids in 19 other nations. *U.S. News & World Report.* Retrieved from https://www.usnews.com/news/best-countries/articles/2018-01-11/us-has-highest-child-mortality-rate-of-20-rich-countries

2   Citizens Commission on Human Rights International. (2017). Number of children and adolescents taking psychiatric drugs in the U.S. CCHR International, The Mental Health Watchdog. Retrieved from www.cchrint.org/psychiatric-drugs/children-on-psychiatric-drugs

3   Salters, J.N. (2017, December 6). 35 Maya Angelou quotes that changed my life. HuffPost. Retrieved from https://www.huffpost.com/entry/35-maya-angelou-quotes-th_b_5412166

4   Institute for Vaccine Safety at Johns Hopkins University. (2019). Vaccine excipient summary [PDF file]. Baltimore, MD: Johns Hopkins University. Retrieved from https://www.cdc.gov/vaccines/pubs/pinkbook/downloads/appendices/B/excipient-table-2.pdf

5   Immunization Action Coalition. (2019). Food and Drug Administration: Package Inserts & FDA Product Approvals. Retrieved from http://www.immunize.org/fda/

6   National Vaccine Information Center. (1982-2019). The National Childhood Vaccine Injury Act of 1986. Sterling, VA: National Vaccine Information Center. Retrieved from https://www.nvic.org/injury-compensation/origihanlaw.aspx

7   Roundtable on Environmental Health Sciences, Research, and Medicine; Board on Population Health and Public Health Practice; Institute of Medicine. (2014). Identifying and Reducing Environmental Health Risks of Chemicals in Our Society: Workshop Summary. Washington, D.C.: National Academies Press (U.S,). Retrieved from https://www.ncbi.nlm.nih.gov/books/NBK268889/

8   Trager, Rebecca. (2016, June 14). New toxic chemical law can improve safety and the environment. Scientific American. Retrieved from https://www.scientificamerican.com/article/new-toxic-chemical-law-can-improve-safety-and-the-environment/

9   Ibid

10   Environmental Working Group (EWG). (2019). https://www.ewg.org/

11   Roundtable on Environmental Health Sciences, Research, and Medicine; Board on Population Health and Public Health Practice; Institute of Medicine. (2014). Identifying and Reducing Environmental Health Risks of Chemicals in Our Society: Workshop Summary. Washington, D.C.: National Academies Press (U.S,). Retrieved from https://www.ncbi.nlm.nih.gov/books/NBK268889/

12   Trager, Rebecca. (2016, June 14). New toxic chemical law can improve safety and the environment. Scientific American. Retrieved from https://www.scientificamerican.com/article/new-toxic-chemical-law-can-improve-safety-and-the-environment/

13   An amendment to this law was introduced to the U.S. Congress in 2018 but failed to pass; Safe Cosmetics and Personal Care Products Act of 2018, H.R. 6903 — 115th Congress. (2018). Retrieved from https://www.govtrack.us/congress/bills/115/hr6903

14   Product Safety. (2018). BeautyTruth.com. Retrieved from http://www.beautytruth.com/fda

15   Environmental Working Group. (2005, July 14). Body burden: The pollution in Newborns. Environmental Working Group. Retrieved from https://www.ewg.org/research/body-burden-pollution-newborns

16   Breast Cancer Prevention Partners. (2019). Low dose effects and timing of exposures. Retrieved from https://www.bcpp.org/our-work/core-science/

17   Green Science Policy Institute. (2019). Safe kids campaign. Retrieved from https://greensciencepolicy.org/topics/safe-kids-campaign/

18   Chicago Tribune Watchdog. (2012). Playing with fire. Retrieved from https://media.apps.chicagotribune.com/flames/index.html

19   Project TENDR. (2019). Chemicals and pollutants. Retrieved from http://projecttendr.com/chemicals-and-pollutants/

20   Organization That Made the Standard. (2001). Medical surveillance: Formaldehyde (Standard No. 1910.1048 App C). Retrieved from https://www.osha.gov/laws-regs/regulations/standardnumber/1910/1910.1048AppC

21   https://scholar.google.com/scholar?g=bpa+contributing+to+obesity+neurological+and+immune+disorders&hl=en&as_sdt=0&as_vis=1&oi=scholar&sa=X&ei=LwWFUtu9HoWo4APU0ICAAw&ved=0CDcQgQMwAA

22   WebMD. (2005-2019). The facts about bisphenol a. Retrieved from https://www.webmd.com/children/bpa

23   Yang, C., Yaniger, S.I., Jordan, V. C., Klein, D. J., & Bittner, G.D. (2011). Most plastic products release estrogenic chemicals: A potential health problem that can be solved. Environmental Health Perspectives Journal, 119(7), 989–996. https://www.ncbi.nlm.nih.gov/pmc/articles/PMC3222987/

24   Moore, K.L., and Dalley, A.F. (2009). *Clinically Oriented Anatomy* (Sixth Edition). New York, NY: Lippincott Williams and Wilkins.

25   McDonald, J.W., Becker, D., Sadowsky, C.L., Jane, J.A. Sr., Conturo, T.E., & Schultz, L.M. (2002). Late recovery following spinal cord injury: Case report and review of the literature. Journal of Neurosurgery, 97(suppl 2), 252-65. https://www.ncbi.nlm.nih.gov/pubmed/12296690

26   Mercola, J. (2012, February 18). A root canal is a dangerous dental procedure [PDF file]. Retrieved from https://www.hoffmancentre.com/wp-content/uploads/2016/12/Why_A_Root_Canal_is_a_Dangerous_Dental_Procedure.pdf

27   National Research Council. (2006). Fluoride in drinking water: A scientific review of EPA's standards. Washington, D.C.: National Research Council. Retrieved from https://www.nap.edu/read/11571/chapter/11#270

28   National Institute of Dental and Craniofacial Research. (n.d.). The story of fluoridation. Retrieved from https://www.nidcr.nih.gov/health-info/fluoride/the-story-of-fluoridation

29   Meiers, P. (2018). Patents on fluoride rat poison and insecticides. Retrieved from http://www.fluoride-history.de/p-insecticides.htm

30   Fluoride Toxicity Research Collaborative. (n.d.) Index of fluorinated pharmaceuticals. Retrieved from http://www.slweb.org/ftrcfluorinatedpharm.html

31   Maddison, B. (2015). *A User's Guide to Understanding Fallacy, Fraud and Failure.* New Zealand: Bob Maddison.

32   Ibid

33   Hicks, J. (2011, Summer). Pipe dreams: America's fluoride controversy. Retrieved from https://www.sciencehistory.org/distillations/magazine/pipe-dreams-americas-fluoride-controversy

34   Seavey, J. (2005). Water fluoridation and crime in America. Fluoride 38(1), 11-22. https://pdfs.semanticscholar.org/d0e6/a4b5f474375e800aa9b50422fcd71253f664.pdf

35   Ibid

36   Edwards, R. (2017, October 15). Is fluoride bad for you? It's not just in the water. Retrieved from https://draxe.com/is-fluoride-bad-for-you/

37   Mercola, J. (2014, March 22). First case study to show direct link between Alzheimer's and aluminum toxicity [Blog post. Retrieved from https://articl]es.mercola.com/sites/articles/archive/2014/03/22/aluminum-toxicity-alzheimers.aspx

38   Mercola, J. (2018, April 10). Cell phone radiation linked to brain and heart tumors [Blog post]. Retrieved from https://articles.mercola.com/sites/articles/archive/2018/04/10/cellphone-radiation-linked-to-brain-heart-tumors.aspx

39   Carlson, K. (2019, March 28). Turned off: Sprint shuts down cell tower at Ripon school over parents' cancer concerns. The Modesto Bee. Retrieved from https://www.modbee.com/news/article228538324.html

40   WorldHealth.net. (2019, March 23). Experts warn about the side effects of 5G requiring 20.000 satellites [Blog post]. Retrieved from https://www.worldhealth.net/news/experts-warn-about-side-effects-5g-requiring-20000-satellites/

41   Mercola, J. (2019, April 22). Cell tower removed from schoolyard due to cluster of cancer cases [Blog post]. Retrieved from https://articles.mercola.com/sites/articles/archive/2019/04/16/cell-tower-emf-radiation.aspx

42   Medrut, F. (2017). 25 Nikola Tesla quotes to become the inventor of your dreams. Goalcast. Retrieved from https://www.goalcast.com/2017/12/20/25-nikola-tesla-quotes/

43   Dispenza, J. (2017, February 17). What does the spike in the Schumann resonance mean? [Blog post] Retrieved from https://drjoedispenza.net/blog/consciousness/what-does-the-spike-in-the-schumann-resonance-mean/

44   Ibid

45   H2O Labs. (n.d.). Respected health & wellness professionals agree - Distilled water is the best water to drink. Retrieved from http://www.h2olabs.com/t-doctor-recommended-water-distillers.aspx

46   Drugs in the water (2011, June). Drugs in the water. Harvard Health Letter. Retrieved from https://www.health.harvard.edu/newsletter_article/drugs-in-the-water

47   Karelian Heritage. (n.d.) Shungite water [PDF file]. Retrieved from https://karelianheritage.com/image/shungitepictures/for-articles/Shungite-Water.pdf

48   Fluoride Action Network. (n.d.). Pineal gland. Retrieved from https://fluoridealert.org/issues/health/pineal-gland/

49   Akbar, S. (2012, January 21). Tulsi can detoxify fluoridated water. Retrieved from http://fluoridealert.org/news/tulsi-can-detoxify-fluoridated-water/

50   Sircus, M. (2011, November 15). Iodine protects fluoride toxicity. Retrieved from https://drsircus.com/iodine/iodine-protects-fluoride-toxicity/

51   MintPress News Desk. (2015, October 5). How hemp can clean up radiation from Fukushima nuclear disaster. Retrieved from https://www.mintpressnews.com/how-hemp-can-can-clean-up-radiation-from-fukushima-nuclear-disaster/210098/

52   Null, G. (2003). *The Complete Encyclopedia of Natural Healing: A Comprehensive A-Z Listing of Common Chronic Illnesses and their Proven Natural Treatments.* Stamford, CT: Bottom Line Books.

53   Axe, J. (2018, January 11). 10 researched benefits of chiropractic adjustments. Retrieved from https://draxe.com/10-researched-benefits-chiropractic-adjustments

54   Mars, B., & Fielder, C. (2015). *The Country Almanac of Home Remedies: Time-tested and Almost Forgotten Wisdom for Treating Common Ailments, Aches, and Pains Quickly and Naturally.* Birmingham, AL: Sweet Water Press.

55   Mercola, J. (2017, March 01). Study: Vitamin D is more effective than flu vaccine. Retrieved from https://healthimpactnews.com/2017/study-vitamin-d-is-more-effective-than-flu-vaccine/

56   Lindequist, U., Neidermeyer, T., & Julich, W. (2005). The pharmacological potential of mushrooms. Evidence-Based Complementary and Alternative Medicine, 2(3), 285-299. https://www.hindawi.com/journals/ecam/2005/906016/abs/

57   Ren, P., Ren, X., Cheng, L., & Xu, L. (2018). Frankincense, pine needle and geranium essential oils suppress tumor progression through the regulation of the AMPK/mTOR pathway in breast cancer. Oncology Reports,39(1), 129-137. https://www.spandidos-publications.com/or/39/1/129

58   Syrovets, T., Büchele, B., Krauss, C., Laumonnier, Y., & Simmet, T. (2005). Acetyl-boswellic acids inhibit lipopolysaccharide-mediated TNF-α induction in monocytes by direct interaction with IκB kinases. The Journal of Immunology, 174(1), 498-506. http://www.jimmunol.org/content/174/1/498

59   Villegas, H. (2017, May 6). 7 Insane things you must know about using frankincense essential oil (why it should be in your home!) [Blog post]. Retrieved from https://www.healingharvesthomestead.com/home/2017/4/9/insane-things-you-must-know-about-using-frankincense-essential-oil

60   Axe, J. (n.d.). 10 lavender oil benefits for both major diseases and minor ailments. Retrieved from https://draxe.com/lavender-oil-benefits/

61   Ireland, D. J., Greay, S. J., Hooper, C. M., Kissick, H. T., Filion, P., Riley, T. V., & Beilharz, M. W. (2012, August). Topically applied Melaleuca alternifolia (tea tree) oil causes direct anti-cancer cytotoxicity in subcutaneous tumour bearing mice. Journal of Dermatological Science, 67(2), 120-129. https://www.ncbi.nlm.nih.gov/pubmed/22727730

62   Press, Althea (2014). *The Practical Herbal Medicine Handbook: Your Quick Reference Guide to Healing Herbs and Remedies.* New York, NY: Fall River Press.

63   Mars, B., & Fiedler, C. (2015). *The Country Almanac of Home Remedies: Time-tested and Almost Forgotten Wisdom for Treating Hundreds of Common Ailments, Aches, and Pains Quickly and Naturally.* Birmingham, AL: Sweet Water Press.

64   Axe, J. (2018, July 6). 9 Echinacea benefits from colds to cancer. Retrieved from https://draxe.com/echinacea-benefits/

65   Press, Althea (2014). *The Practical Herbal Medicine Handbook: Your Quick Reference Guide to Healing Herbs and Remedies.* New York, NY: Fall River Press.

66   Link, R. (2019, July 10). Elderberry: Natural medicine for colds, flus, allergies and more. Retrieved from https://draxe.com/elderberry/

67   Press, Althea (2014). *The Practical Herbal Medicine Handbook: Your Quick Reference Guide to Healing Herbs and Remedies.* New York, NY: Fall River Press.

68   Patiry, M. (2018, March 30). 10 antiviral herbs to naturally fight infection and how to use them [Blog post]. Retrieved from https://blog.paleohacks.com/antiviral-herbs/#

69   Press, Althea (2014). *The Practical Herbal Medicine Handbook: Your Quick Reference Guide to Healing Herbs and Remedies.* New York, NY: Fall River Press.

70   Montana, S. (2009). Umcka stops the flu and respiratory infections [Blog post]. Retrieved from https://healthyfoodandlife.blogspot.com/2009/08/health-benefits-of-umcka-stops-viral.html?spref=pi

71   Morice, A.H., Marshall, A.E., Higgins, K.S., & Grattan, T.J. (1994, October 01). Effect of inhaled menthol on citric acid induced cough in normal subjects. Thorax, 1994(49),1024-1026. http://thorax.bmj.com/content/49/10/1024.long

72   Press, Althea (2014). *The Practical Herbal Medicine Handbook: Your Quick Reference Guide to Healing Herbs and Remedies.* New York, NY: Fall River Press.

73   Jayakumar, M., & Ignacimuthu, S. (2006, November 30). In vitro antibacterial activity of some plant essential oils. BMC Complementary and Alternative Medicine: The official journal of the International Society for Complementary Medicine Research (ISCMR), 2006(6), 39. https://bmccomplementalternmed.biomedcentral.com/articles/10.1186/1472-6882-6-39

74   Klenner, F. (1994, July). The treatment of poliomyelitis and other virus diseases with vitamin C. Retrieved from http://www.whale.to/m/measles.html

75   Committee on Infection Diseases. (1993, May 1). Vitamin A treatment of measles. Pediatrics, 91(5). Retrieved from http://pediatrics.aappublications.org/content/91/5/1014

76   Friedman, A., & Sklan, D. (1993, January 1). Vitamin A and Immunity. In: Klurfeld D.M. (eds) Nutrition and Immunology. Human Nutrition (A Comprehensive Treatise). Boston, MA: Springer. Retrieved from https://link.springer.com/chapter/10.1007/978-1-4615-2900-2_9

77   Axe, J. (n.d.). 10 lavender oil benefits for both major diseases and minor ailments. Retrieved from https://draxe.com/lavender-oil-benefits/

78   Press, Althea (2014). *The Practical Herbal Medicine Handbook: Your Quick Reference Guide to Healing Herbs and Remedies.* New York, NY: Fall River Press.

79   Ibid

80   Ibid

81   23 Home Remedies to Get Rid of Mumps. (2018, January 24). Home Remedy Hacks. Retrieved from https://www.homeremedyhacks.com/23-home-remedies-get-rid-mumps/

82   Press, Althea (2014). *The Practical Herbal Medicine Handbook: Your Quick Reference Guide to Healing Herbs and Remedies.* New York, NY: Fall River Press.

83   Ibid

84   Thompson, J., & Camp, E. (2017). *The Unvaccinated Child: A Treatment Guide for Parents and Caregivers.* Norman, OK: Vital Health Publishing.

85   Ibid

86   Barr, T. (2000, August 8). US6514487B1. Foam and gel oat protein complex and method of use. Retrieved from https://patents.google.com/patent/US6514487B1/en

87   Thompson, J., & Camp, E. (2017). *The Unvaccinated Child: A Treatment Guide for Parents and Caregivers.* Norman, OK: Vital Health Publishing.

88   Press, Althea (2014). *The Practical Herbal Medicine Handbook: Your Quick Reference Guide to Healing Herbs and Remedies.* New York, NY: Fall River Press.

89   Jayakumar, M., & Ignacimuthu, S. (2006, November 30). In vitro antibacterial activity of some plant essential oils. BMC Complementary and Alternative Medicine: The official journal of the International Society for Complementary Medicine Research (ISCMR), 2006(6), 39. https://bmccomplementalternmed.biomedcentral.com/articles/10.1186/1472-6882-6-39

90   Mihalovic, D. (2016, March 24). The REAL Truth About The Tetanus Vaccine: It Isn't Protecting You From Getting Sick! Retrieved from http://www.healthy-holistic-living.com/tetanus-vaccine-truth.html

91   Humphries, S. (2017, October 17). Sodium ascorbate/ vitamin C treatment of whooping cough. Retrieved from http://drsuzanne.net/2017/10/sodium-ascorbate-vitamin-c-treatment-of-whooping-cough-suzanne-humphries-md/

92   Ormerod, M. J., & Unkauf, B. M. (1937, August). Ascorbic acid (vitamin C) treatment of whooping cough. Canadian Medical Association Journal, 37(2), 134-136. https://www.ncbi.nlm.nih.gov/pmc/articles/PMC1562195/

93   Morice, A.H.., Marshall, A.E.., Higgins, K.S., & Grattan, T.J. (1994, October 01). Effect of inhaled menthol on citric acid induced cough in normal subjects. Thorax, 1994(49),1024-1026. http://thorax.bmj.com/content/49/10/1024.long

94   Thompson, J., & Camp, E. (2017). *The Unvaccinated Child: A Treatment Guide for Parents and Caregivers.* Norman, OK: Vital Health Publishing, p. 55

95   Press, Althea (2014). *The Practical Herbal Medicine Handbook: Your Quick Reference Guide to Healing Herbs and Remedies.* New York, NY: Fall River Press.

96   Humphries, S. (2017, October 17). Sodium ascorbate/ vitamin C treatment of whooping cough. Retrieved from http://drsuzanne.net/2017/10/sodium-ascorbate-vitamin-c-treatment-of-whooping-cough-suzanne-humphries-md/

97   Press, Althea (2014). *The Practical Herbal Medicine Handbook: Your Quick Reference Guide to Healing Herbs and Remedies.* New York, NY: Fall River Press.

98   Mendelsohn, R. S. (1987). *How to raise a healthy child-- in spite of your doctor.* New York: Ballantine, pp. 73-88.

99   1) Mendelsohn, R. S. (1987). *How to Raise a Healthy Child - In Spite of Your Doctor.* New York: Ballantine.

100   Top 10 Hippocrates Quotes. (2019.) Brainy Quote. Retrieved from https://www.brainyquote.com/lists/authors/top_10_hippocrates_quotes

101   Samuelson, G. L., (2018). *A Journey of Discovery into Redox Signaling Biology.* Deep Lake Media.

102   Aquilano, K., Baldelli, S., & Ciriolo M. R., (2014, August 26). Glutathione: New roles in redox signaling for an old antioxidant. Frontiers in Pharmacology, 5, 196. https://www.ncbi.nlm.nih.gov/pubmed/25206336

103   Wu, G., Fang, Y., Yang, S., Lupton, J. R., & Turner, N. D. (2004, March 01). Glutathione metabolism and its implications for health. Journal of Nutrition, 134(3), 489-492. https://www.ncbi.nlm.nih.gov/pubmed/14988435

104   Morse, R. (2004). *The Detox Miracle Sourcebook.* Chino Valley, AZ: Kalindi Press.

105   Ibid.

106   Ehret, A. (1953/1994). *Mucusless Diet Healing System.* Ardsley, NY: Ehret Literature Publishing Co. Inc.

107   Morse, R. (2004). *The Detox Miracle Sourcebook.* Chino Valley, AZ: Kalindi Press.

108   Martin, N., & Montagne, R. (2017, May 12). U.S. has the worst rate of maternal deaths in the developed world. NPR. Retrieved from https://www.npr.org/2017/05/12/528098789/u-s-has-the-worst-rate-of-maternal-deaths-in-the-developed-world

109   Ibid

110   Adams, K. M., Lindell, K. C., Kohlmeier, M., & Zeisel, S. H. (2008). Status of nutrition education in medical schools. American Journal of Clinical Nutrition, 83(4), 941S-944

S. Retrieved from https://www.ncbi.nlm.nih.gov/pmc/articles/PMC2430660/

111   Miller, N. Z., & Goldman, G. S. (2011). Infant mortality rates regressed against number of vaccine doses routinely given: Is there a biochemical or synergistic toxicity? Human & Experimental Toxicology, 30(9), 1420-1428. Retrieved from https://www.ncbi.nlm.nih.gov/pmc/articles/PMC3170075/

112   Goldman, G. S., & Miller, N. (2012). Relative trends in hospitalizations and mortality among infants by the number of vaccine doses and age, based on the vaccine adverse event reporting system (VAERS), 1990–2010. Human and Experimental Toxicology,31(10), 1012-1021. Retrieved from https://www.ncbi.nlm.nih.gov/pmc/articles/PMC3547435/pdf/10.1177_0960327112440111.pdf.

113   American College of Obstetricians and Gynecologists. (2015) Frequently asked questions for pregnant women concerning TDaP vaccine [Tear Pad]. Washington, DC: American College of Obstetricians and Gynecologists. Retrieved from https://www.acog.org/-/media/Departments/Immunization/Tdap-Vaccine-Mailing/Tear-pad-FAQTDAP.pdf

114   GlaxoSmithKline Biologicals. (n.d.) Package Insert - Infanrix [Brochure]. Research Triangle Park, NC: Author. Retrieved from https://www.fda.gov/downloads/biologicsbloodvaccines/vaccines/approvedproducts/ucm124514.pdf

115   Sukumaran, L., McCarthy, N.L., Kharbanda, E.O., Vazquez-Benitez, G., Lipkind, H.S., Jackson, L., Klein, N.P., Naleway, A.L., McClure, D.L., Hechter, R.C., Kawai, A.T., Glanz, J.M., & Weintraub, E.S. (2018). Infant hospitalizations and mortality after maternal vaccination. Pediatrics, 141(3). https://pediatrics.aappublications.org/content/141/3/e20173310

116   Cherry, J. (2019). The 112-year odyssey of pertussis and pertussis vaccines-mistakes made and implications for the future. Journal of the American Pediatric Disease Society, February 22. https://www.ncbi.nlm.nih.gov/pubmed/30793754

117   Warfel, J. M., Zimmerman, L. I., & Merkel, T. J. (2016). Comparison of three whole-cell pertussis vaccines in the baboon model of pertussis. Clinical and Vaccine Immunology, 47-54. https://cvi.asm.org/content/23/1/47

118   Sanofi Pasteurs. (n.d.). Package insert - 450/477 Fluzone® Quadrivalent [Brochure]. Research Swiftwater, PA. Retrieved from https://www.fda.gov/downloads/biologicsbloodvaccines/vaccines/approvedproducts/ucm356094.pdf

119   Jefferson, T, Di Pietrantonj, C, Rivetti, A, Bawazeer, G.A., Al Ansary, L.A., & Ferroni, E. (2010). Vaccines for preventing influenza in healthy adults. Cochrane Database of Systematic Reviews, 7(CD001269). https://www.cochranelibrary.com/cdsr/doi/10.1002/14651858.CD001269.pub4/abstract

120   Donahue, E. (2017). Association of spontaneous abortion with receipt of inactivated influenza vaccine containing H1N1pdm09 in 2010-11 and 2011-12. Vaccine, 35(40), 5314-5322. https://www.ncbi.nlm.nih.gov/pubmed/28917295

121   Cowling, B. J., Fang, V. J., Nishiura, H., Chan, K.-H., Ng, S., Ip, D. K. M., ... Peiris, J. S. M. (2012). Increased risk of noninfluenza respiratory virus infections associated with receipt of inactivated influenza vaccine. Clinical Infectious Diseases: An Official Publication of the Infectious Diseases Society of America, 54(12), 1778–1783. https://academic.oup.com/cid/article/54/12/1778/455098

122   Skowronski, D.M., De Serres, G., Crowcroft, N.S., Janjua, N.Z., Boulianne, N., Hottes, T.S., et al. (2010) Association between the 2008–09 seasonal influenza vaccine and pandemic H1N1 illness during Spring–Summer 2009: Four observational studies from Canada. PLoS Med 7(4): e1000258. Retrieved from https://doi.org/10.1371/journal.pmed.1000258

123   Lippi, G., & Franchini, M. (2011). Vitamin K in neonates: Facts and myths. Blood Transfusion,4-9. https://www.ncbi.nlm.nih.gov/pmc/articles/PMC3021393/

124   Merck & Co., Inc. (n.d.). Package Insert - AquaMEPHYTON [Brochure]. Whitehouse Station, NJ: Merck & Co., Inc. Retrieved from https://www.accessdata.fda.gov/drugsatfda_docs/label/2003/012223Orig1s039Lbl.pdf

125   Blackmon, E. (2003). Controversies concerning vitamin K and the newborn. Pediatrics,112(1). Retrieved from https://pediatrics.aappublications.org/content/112/1/191

126   National Vaccine Information Center. (n.d.). Hepatitis b disease & vaccine information. Retrieved from https://www.nvic.org/Vaccines-and-Diseases/Hepatitis-B.aspx

127   Kolata, G. (1991, March 1). U.S. panel urges that all children be vaccinated for hepatitis b. The New York Times. Retrieved from https://www.nytimes.com/1991/03/01/us/us-panel-urges-that-all-children-be-vaccinated-for-hepatitis-b.html

128   European Consensus Group on Hepatitis B Immunity. (2000, February 12). Consensus statement: Are booster immunisations needed for lifelong hepatitis b immunity? The Lancet,355(9203), 561-565. https://www.thelancet.com/journals/lancet/article/PIIS0140-6736(99)07239-6/fulltext

129   Handley, J. (2018, July 02). New study: Hep b vaccine "may have adverse implications for brain development and cognition." [Blog post]. Retrieved from https://jbhandleyblog.com/home/2018/7/2/hepbthree

130   Tarakji, B., Ashok, N., Alakeel, R., Azzeghaibi, S., Umair, A., Darwish, S., Mahmoud, R., & Elkhatat, E. (2014, November). Hepatitis B vaccination and associated oral manifestations: A non-systematic review of literature and case reports. Annals of Medical and Health Science Research 4(6):829-36. https://www.ncbi.nlm.nih.gov/m/pubmed/25506472/

131   Informed Choice Washington. (2017, September). Pregnancy & vaccination. Retrieved from https://www.informedchoicewa.org/vaccination-during-pregnancy

132   Children's Health Defense. (2019, February 12). FDA admits that government is recommending untested, unlicensed vaccines for pregnant women. Children's Health Defense. Retrieved from https://childrenshealthdefense.org/news/fda-admits-that-government-is-recommending-untested-unlicensed-vaccines-for-pregnant-women/

133   Top 10 Lao Tzu quotes. (2019). Brainy Quote. Retrieved from https://www.brainyquote.com/lists/authors/top_10_lao_tzu_quotes

134   Turner, J. (2012) *Vaccine Epidemic: How Corporate Greed, Biased Science, and Coercive Government Threaten Our Human Rights, Our Health, and Our Children (Expanded Third Edition).* New York, NY: Skyhorse.

135   Health Resources and Services Administration. (2019, June). National vaccine injury compensation program. Retrieved from https://www.hrsa.gov/vaccine-compensation/index.html

136   National Vaccine Information Center. (2019). Report vaccine reactions. It's the law! Retrieved from https://www.nvic.org/reportreaction.aspx

137   National Vaccine Information Center. (2019) State vaccine requirements. Retrieved from www.nvic.org/vaccine-laws/state-vaccine-requirements.aspx

138   Ibid

139   National Vaccine Information Center. (2019). Vaccine exemptions FAQs. Retrieved from www.nvic.org/faqs/vaccine-exemptions.aspx

140   Ibid

141   Wrangham, T. (2011, February 1). College bound - navigating vaccine choices. National Vaccine Information Center. Retrieved from .https://www.vic.org/NVIC-Vaccine-News/February-2011/College-Bound---Navigating-Vaccine-Choices.aspx

142   Supreme court gives big pharmaceuticals a vaccination against lawsuits. (2011, October 27). Pace International Law Review. Retrieved from: pilr.blogs.pace.edu/2011/10/27/supreme-court-gives-big-pharmaceuticals-a-vaccination-against-lawsuits/

143   National Vaccine Information Center. (2019). National Childhood Vaccine Injury Act of 1986. Retrieved from https://www.nvic.org/Vaccine-Laws/1986-Vaccine-Injury-Law.aspx

144   Health Resources and Services Administration. (2019, March). National vaccine injury compensation program. Retrieved from www.hrsa.gov/vaccine-compensation/index.html

145   Turner, J. (2012) *Vaccine Epidemic: How Corporate Greed, Biased Science, and Coercive Government Threaten Our Human Rights, Our Health, and Our Children (Expanded Third Edition).* New York, NY: Skyhorse, pp. 32-32.

146   National Vaccine Information Center. (2019). Report vaccine reactions. It's the law! Retrieved from https://www.nvic.org/reportreaction.aspx.

147   Nuremberg Military Tribunal. (1949). Trials of War Criminals before the Nuremberg Military Tribunals under Control Council Law, No. 10(2). Washington, D.C.: U.S. Government Printing Office.

148   Herbert, C. (2019, April 23). Social media anti-vaccine censorship worries some. Albany Herald. Retrieved from www.albanyherald.com/features/social-media-anti-vaccine-censorship-worries-some/article_9ff76376-65d9-11e9-a138-579408b3b1fa.html

149   Whitney, A. (2015, August) Do not sign the refusal to vaccinate form! Parents Against Mandatory Vaccines. Retrieved from https://parentsaganinstmandatoryvaccines.net/2015/08/18/do-not-sign-the-refusal-to-vaccinate-form/.

150   Revolution for Choice. (2018, December 5). When you absolutely must sign a form, here is a legal way to protect yourself. Retrieved from https//m.facebook.com/notes/revolution-for-choice/when-you-absolutely-must-sign-a-form-here-is-a-legal-way-to-protect-yourself/147359595671635/

151   Ibid

152   Ibid

153   Parents Against Mandatory Vaccines. (2017). The vaccination notice. Retrieved from https://parentsaganinstmandatoryvaccines.net/the-vaccination-notice/.

154   Revolution for Choice. (2018, December 5). When you absolutely must sign a form, here is a legal way to protect yourself. Retrieved from https//m.facebook.com/notes/revolution-for-choice/when-you-absolutely-must-sign-a-form-here-is-a-legal-way-to-protect-yourself/147359595671635/

155   Whitney, A. (2015, January). So, you've signed the refusal to vaccinate document? Parents Against Mandatory Vaccines. Retrieved from https://parentsaganinstmandatoryvaccines.net/2015/01/26/so-youve-signed-the-refusal-to-vaccinate-document/.

156   Modern Alternative Mama. (2019, March). A script for dealing with doctors that coerce you to vaccinate. Retrieved from https://modernalternativemama. com/2019/03/16/a-script-for-dealing-with-doctors-that-coerce-you-to-vaccinate/

157   Jaxen, J. (2016, May). Nurse whistleblower: Hospitals vaccinating patients by force without their knowledge. Vaccine Impact. Retrieved from https://vaccineimpact. com/2016/nurse-whistleblower-hospitals-vaccinating-patients-by-force-without-their-knowledge/

158   Caceres, M., and Parpia, R. (2018). Biologics r vaccines: Beware of 'informed consent.' The Vaccine Reaction. Retrieved from https://thevaccinereaction. org/2018/01/biologics-r-vaccines-beware-of-informed-consent/

159   Vaccine Truth Movement. (2019) Vaccine safety - are we really safe? Retrieved from http://www.arevaccinessafe.org/are-vaccines-safe/

160   Children's Health Defense. (2019). Too many sick children. Children's Health Defense. Retrieved from childrenshealthdefense.org/too-many-sick-children/

161   Centers for Disease Control and Prevention. (2018). Frequently asked questions about estimated flu burden. Retrieved from https://www.cdc.gov/flu/about/disease/ us_flu-related_deaths.htm

162   McNeil, D.G. Jr. (2018, October 1). Over 80,000 Americans died of flu last winter, highest toll in years. New York Times. Retrieved from https://www.nytimes. com/2018/10/01/health/flu-deaths-vaccine.html

163   National Foundation for Infectious Diseases. (2018). 2018 NFID influenza/ pneumococcal news conference. Retrieved from http://www.nfid.org/newsroom/ news-conferences/2018-nfid-influenza-pneumococcal-news-conference

164   Centers for Disease Control and Prevention. (2018). Frequently asked questions about estimated flu burden. Retrieved from https://www.cdc.gov/flu/about/disease/ us_flu-related_deaths.htm

165   Centers for Disease Control and Prevention. (2018). Diagnosing flu. Retrieved from https://www.cdc.gov/flu/about/qa/testing.htm

166   Centers for Disease Control and Prevention. (2018). Frequently asked questions about estimated flu burden. Retrieved from https://www.cdc.gov/flu/about/burden/faq. htm

167   Centers for Disease Control and Prevention. (2018). Summary of the 2017-2018 influenza season. Retrieved from https://www.cdc.gov/flu/about/season/flu-season-2017-2018.htm

168   Ibid

169   Jefferson, T., Rivetti, A., Di Pietrantonj, C., Demicheli, V., & Ferroni, E. (2012). Vaccines for preventing influenza in healthy children. Cochrane Database of Systematic Reviews 2012(8), Art. No.: CD004879. https://www.cochranelibrary.com/cdsr/ doi/10.1002/14651858.CD004879.pub4/full

170   Centers for Disease Control and Prevention. (2017). Influenza (flu) vaccine safety. Retrieved from https://www.cdc.gov/flu/protect/vaccine/vaccinesafety.htm

171   Milani, K. & Duffy, D. (2019, February). Profits over patients: How the rules of our economy encourage the pharmaceutical industry's extractive behavior [PDF file]. Retrieved from http://rooseveltinstitute.org/wp-content/uploads/2019/02/RI_ Profit-Over-Patients_brief_021319-1.pdf

172   U.S. Food and Drug Administration. (2014). Types of applications. Retrieved from https://www.fda.gov/Drugs/DevelopmentApprovalProcess/ HowDrugsareDevelopedandApproved/ApprovalApplications/default.htm

173   U.S. Food and Drug Administration. (2019). FDA's Critical Role in Ensuring Supply of Influenza Vaccine. Retrieved from https://www.fda.gov/ForConsumers/ConsumerUpdates/ucm336267.htm

174   U.S. Food and Drug Administration. (2018). Influenza virus vaccine safety and availability. Retrieved from https://www.fda.gov/biologicsbloodvaccines/safetyavailability/vaccinesafety/ucm110288.htm

175   VAERS table of reportable events following vaccination [PDF]. (n.d.). Retrieved from https://vaers.hhs.gov/docs/VAERS_Table_of_Reportable_Events_Following_Vaccination.pdf

176   Jefferson, T., Rivetti, A., Di Pietrantonj, C., Demicheli, V., & Ferroni, E. (2012). Vaccines for preventing influenza in healthy children. Cochrane Database of Systematic Reviews 2012(8), Art. No.: CD004879. https://www.ncbi.nlm.nih.gov/pubmed/22895945

177   Ibid

178   Ibid

179   American Thoracic Society. (2009, May). Children who get flu vaccine have three times risk of hospitalization for flu, study suggests. ScienceDaily. Retrieved from www.sciencedaily.com/releases/2009/05/090519172045.htm

180   Cowling, B. J., Fang, V. J., Nishiura, H., Chan, K.-H., Ng, S., Ip, D. K. M., ... Peiris, J. S. M. (2012). Increased risk of noninfluenza respiratory virus infections associated with receipt of inactivated influenza vaccine. Clinical Infectious Diseases: An Official Publication of the Infectious Diseases Society of America, 54(12), 1778–1783. https://academic.oup.com/cid/article/54/12/1778/455098

181   Bodewes, R., Fraaij, P. L. A., Geelhoed-Mieras, M. M., van Baalen, C. A., Tiddens, H. A. W. M., van Rossum, A. M. C., ... Rimmelzwaan, G. F. (2011). Annual vaccination against influenza virus hampers development of virus-specific CD8+ T cell immunity in children. Journal of Virology, 85(22), 11995–12000. https://jvi.asm.org/content/85/22/11995

182   Zhou, W., Pool, V., Iskander, J.K., English-Bullard, R., Ball, R., Wise, R.P., ... Chen, R.T. (2003) Surveillance for safety after immunization: Vaccine adverse event reporting system (VAERS) — United States, 1991-2001. MMWR Surveillance Summary, 52(1);1-24. Retrieved from https://www.cdc.gov/mmwr/preview/mmwrhtml/ss5201a1.htm

183   Neidich, S.D., Green, W.D., Rebeles, J., Karlsson, E.A., Schultz- Cherry, S., Noah, T.L., & Beck, M.A. (2017). Increased risk of influenza among vaccinated adults who are obese, International Journal of Obesity 41(9), 1324-1330. https://www.ncbi.nlm.nih.gov/pubmed/28584297

184   Ayling, K., Fairclough, L., Tighe, P., Todd, I., Halliday, V., Garibaldi, J., & Vedhara, K. (2018). Positive mood on the day of influenza vaccination predicts vaccine effectiveness: A prospective observational cohort study. Brain, Behavior, and Immunity, 67(0), 314-323. https://www.ncbi.nlm.nih.gov/pubmed/28923405

185   Li-Kim-Moy, J., Yin, J.K., Rashid, H., Khandaker, G., King, C., Wood, N., & Booy, R. (2015). Systematic review of fever, febrile convulsions and serious adverse events following administration of inactivated trivalent influenza vaccines in children. EuroSurveillance 20(24).

186   Janjua, N.Z., Skowronski, D.M., Hottes, T.S., Osei, W., Adams, E., Petric, M., ... Bowering, D. (2010). Seasonal influenza vaccine and increased risk of pandemic A/H1N1-related illness: First detection of the association in British Columbia,

Canada. Clinical Infectious Diseases, 51(9), 1017–1027. https://www.ncbi.nlm.nih.gov/pubmed/20887210

187   Centers for Disease Control. (2018). 2018-2019 ACIP Background: Safety of influenza vaccines. Retrieved from https://www.cdc.gov/flu/professionals/acip/2018-2019/background/safety-vaccines.htm

188   For more information about the herd immunity theory, see the publications of Tetyana Obukhanych and Suzanne Humphries.

189   Han, J.M., Patterson, S.J., Speck, M., Ehses, J.A., & Levings, M.K. (2014). Insulin inhibits IL-10–mediated regulatory T-cell function: Implications for obesity. The Journal of Immunology 192(2), 623-629. https://www.jimmunol.org/content/early/2013/12/08/jimmunol.1302181

190   Watson, N.F., Buchwald, D., Delrow J.J., Altemeier, W.A., Vitiello, M.V., Pack, A.I., ... Gharib, S.A. (2017). Transcriptional signatures of sleep duration discordance in monozygotic twins. Sleep 40(1), zsw019. https://academic.oup.com/sleep/article/40/1/zsw019/2952682

191   Jørgensen, L., Gøtzsche, P.C., & Jefferson, T. (2018). The Cochrane HPV vaccine review was incomplete and ignored important evidence of bias. BMJ Evidence-Based Medicine 2018(23),165-168. https://ebm.bmj.com/content/23/5/165

192   Bastian, H. (2019, April 29). Should we trust meta-analyses with meta-conflicts of interest? [Blog post]. Retrieved from https://blogs.plos.org/absolutely-maybe/2019/04/28/should-we-trust-meta-analyses-with-meta-conflicts-of-interest/

193   Marcus, A., & Oransky, I. (2018, September 16). Turmoil erupts over expulsion from leading evidence-based medicine group. Retrieved from https://www.statnews.com/2018/09/16/expulsion-cochrane-peter-gotzsche-medicine/

194   Vesper, I. (2018, September 17). Mass resignation guts board of prestigious Cochrane Collaboration. Nature. Retrieved from https://www.nature.com/articles/d41586-018-06727-0

195   Merck & Co., Inc. (n.d.). Gardasil Package Insert. Retrieved from https://www.fda.gov/files/vaccines,%20blood%20&%20biologics/published/Package-Insert---Gardasil.pdf

196   Tarsell, Emily. (n.d.). Gardasil and Unexplained Deaths.com. Retrieved from http://www.gardasil-and-unexplained-deaths.com/

197   What Is Glutathione and How Is It Good For Your Health? (2014, December 10). Retrieved from https://healthynews24.com/health-benefits-of-glutathione/

198   Walia, Arjun. (2016, April 12). Lead Developer Of HPV Vaccines Comes Clean To Warn Parents & Young Girls. Collective Evolution. Retrieved from https://www.collective-evolution.com/2016/04/12/lead-developer-of-hpv-vaccines-comes-clean-to-warn-parents-young-girls/

199   Ibid

200   Madatyan, Marine. (2017, December 18). 700 Women in Columbia Vaccinated with Gardasil Sue Merck for $160 Million: Researcher Advices Girls in Armenia to Understand the Risks. HETQ. Retrieved from https://hetq.am/en/article/84400

201   Carolan, Mary. (2015, November 2). Court told of 'horrendous adverse effects' of HPV vaccine. Irish Times. Retrieved from https://www.irishtimes.com/news/crime-and-law/courts/high-court/court-told-of-horrendous-adverse-effects-of-hpv-vaccine-1.2414549

202   Centers for Disease Control. (2019). Immunization schedules. Retrieved from https://www.cdc.gov/vaccines/schedules/index.html.

203   Phrma Docs. (2016). Vaccines in Development. Medicines in Development: Vaccines [PDF file]. Retrieved from http://phrma-docs.phrma.org/sites/default/files/pdf/medicines-in-development-drug-list-vaccines.pdf

204   Sound Choice Pharmaceutical Institute. Theresa Deisher, Ph.D. Autism One. 2013. "Autism Disorder Changepoints and Environmental Triggers."

205   Center for Disease Control and Prevention. (2018). Vaccine Excipient & Media Summary. Retrieved at https://www.cdc.gov/vaccines/pubs/pinkbook/downloads/appendices/B/excipient-table-2.pdf

206   Sound Choice Pharmaceutical Institute. Theresa Deisher, Ph.D. Autism One. 2013. "Autism Disorder Changepoints and Environmental Triggers."

207   International Agency for Research on Cancer. (2006). Formaldehyde. Retrieved from https://monographs.iarc.fr/wp-content/uploads/2018/06/mono100F-29.pdf

208   Center for Disease Control and Prevention. (2018). Vaccine Excipient & Media Summary. Retrieved from https://www.cdc.gov/vaccines/pubs/pinkbook/downloads/appendices/B/excipient-table-2.pdf

209   GlaxoSmithKline. (n.d.). Infanrix Manufacturer Insert. Carcinogenesis, Mutagenesis, Impairment of Fertility [PDF] Line 324-325. Retrieved from https://www.fda.gov/media/75157/download

210   Merck & Co., Inc. (Revised December 2018). Recombivax Manufacturer Insert (Recombinant). 6.2 Post-Marketing Experience. Retrieved from https://www.fda.gov/media/74274/download

211   Shaw, C.A., Seneff, S., Kette, S.D., Tomljenovic, L., Oller, J.W. Jr., & Davidson, R. (2014, October 2) Aluminum-induced entropy in biological systems: Implications for neurological disease. Journal of Toxicology v2014, 491316. https://www.ncbi.nlm.nih.gov/pmc/articles/PMC4202242/

212   Center for Disease Control and Prevention. (2018). Vaccine Excipient & Media Summary. Retrieved from https://www.cdc.gov/vaccines/pubs/pinkbook/downloads/appendices/B/excipient-table-2.pdf

213   Ibid

214   Haines, A., Kuruvilla, S., & Borchert, M. (2004) Bridging the implementation gap between knowledge and action for health. Bulletin of the World Health Organization 82, 724-732. Retrieved from https://www.who.int/bulletin/volumes/82/10/724.pdf

215   Health Resources and Services Administration. (2019). Vaccine Injury Compensation Data. Retrieved from https://www.hrsa.gov/vaccine-compensation/data/index.html

216   Office of the Law Revision Council. 42 USC Chapter 6A, Subchapter XIX: Vaccines. National Vaccine Program. United States Code. Retrieved from http://uscode.house.gov/view.xhtml?path=/prelim@title42/chapter6A/subchapter19&edition=prelim

217   Committee on the Assessment of Studies of Health Outcomes Related to the Recommended Childhood Immunization Schedule; Board on Population Health and Public Health Practice; Institute of Medicine. (2013). The Childhood Immunization Schedule and Safety: Stakeholder Concerns, Scientific Evidence, and Future Studies. Washington, D.C.: NCBI National Library of Medicine.

218   Pollan, M. (2007). *The Omnivore's Dilemma: A Natural History of Four Meals.* New York City, NY: Penguin.

219   Roseboro, Ken. (2011, March 1). Most "natural" cereals likely to contain GMOs. The Organic & Non-GMO Report. Retrieved from https://non-gmoreport.com/articles/march2011/naturalcerealscontaingmos.php

220   Natural vs. Organic Cereal. (2011, October 11). The Cornucopia Institute. Retrieved from https://www.cornucopia.org/2011/10/natural-vs-organic-cereal/

221   Quick, A.J. (1975). The role of vitamins in hemostasis. Thrombosis et Diathesis Haemorrhagica, 33(2), 191-8.

222   Weston A. Price Foundation. (2005, December 26). Dirty secrets of the food processing industry. Weston A. Price Foundation. Retrieved from https://www.westonaprice.org/health-topics/modern-foods/dirty-secrets-of-the-food-processing-industry/

223   Weston A. Price Foundation. (2000, January 1). Broth is beautiful. Weston A. Price Foundation. Retrieved from https://www.westonaprice.org/health-topics/food-features/broth-is-beautiful/ January 1, 2000

224   Innis, S.M. (2008). Dietary omega 3 acids and the developing brain. Brain Research, 1237, 35-43. https://www.sciencedirect.com/science/article/pii/S0006899308021033?via%3Dihub

225   Besedovsky, L., Lange, T. & Born, J. (20120. Sleep and immune function. Pflügers Archiv - European Journal of Physiology, 463,121. https://doi.org/10.1007/s00424-011-1044-0

226   Irwin, M.R., & Opp, M.R. (2017). Sleep health: Reciprocal regulation of sleep and innate immunity. Neuropsychopharmacology, 42, 129-155. https://www.nature.com/articles/npp2016148

227   Zahl, T., Steinsbekk, S., & Wichstrøm, L. (2017). Physical activity, sedentary behavior, and symptoms of major depression in middle childhood. Pediatrics, 139(2). https://pediatrics.aappublications.org/content/139/2/e20161711..info

228   Radom-Aizik, S. (2017). Immune response to exercise during growth. Human Kinetics Journals, 29(1), 49-52. https://journals.humankinetics.com/doi/10.1123/pes.2017-0003

229   Sothern, M. S., Loftin, M., Suskind, R.M., Udall, J.N., & Blecker, U. (1999). The health benefits of physical activity in children and adolescents: implications for chronic disease prevention. European Journal of Pediatrics, 158(4), 271-274. https://link.springer.com/article/10.1007/s004310051070#citeas

230   Ximenez, C., & Torres, J. (2017). Development of microbiota in infants and its role in maturation of gut mucosa and immunesSystem. Archives of Medical Research,48(8), 666-680. https://doi.org/10.1016/j.arcmed.2017.11.007

231   Brown University. (2018, December 18). Gut microbiome regulates the intestinal immune system. ScienceDaily. Retrieved May 15, 2019 from http://www.sciencedaily.com/releases/2018/12/181218123123.htm

232   Mezouar, S., Chantran, Y., Michel, J., Fabre, A., Dubus, J., Leone, M., Sereme, Y., Mège, J., Ranque, S., Desnues, B., Chanez, P., & Vitte, J. (2018). Microbiome and the immune system: From a healthy steady-state to allergy associated disruption. Human Microbiome Journal, 10, 11-20. https://doi.org/10.1016/j.humic.2018.10.001

233   Campbell-McBride, N., MD. (2012). Gut and Psychology Syndrome. Cambridge, UK: Medinform Publishing.

234   Kural, B. V., Küçük, N., Yücesan, F. B., & Ören, A. (2011). Effects of kale (Brassica oleracea L. var. acephala DC) leaves extracts on the susceptibility of very low and low density lipoproteins to oxidation. Indian Journal of Biochemistry and Biophysics,48(5), 361-364. http://hdl.handle.net/123456789/12946

235   Wendel, L. (2018, May 16). 26 Science-Backed Health Benefits of Kale. Retrieved from https://healthyline.com/health-benefits-of-kale/

236   Pérez-Cano, F. J., Massot-Cladera, M., Franch, À, Castellote, C., & Castell, M. (2013). The effects of cocoa on the immune system. Frontiers in Pharmacology,4. https://doi.org/10.3389/fphar.2013.00071

237   Alton, L. (2016, August 27). Chia seeds boost immune function and protect the heart. Retrieved from https://www.naturalhealth365.com/chia-seeds-heart-health-1850.html

238   Szalay, J. (2014, October 23). Avocados: Health benefits, risks & nutrition facts. Retrieved from https://www.livescience.com/45209-avocado-nutrition-facts.html

239   Axe, J. (2018, August 27). Elderberry: Natural medicine for colds, flus, allergies and more. Retrieved from https://www.circleofdocs.com/elderberry-natural-medicine-for-colds-flus-allergies-more/

240   Tiralongo, E., Wee, S., & Lea, R. (2016). Elderberry supplementation reduces cold duration and symptoms in air-travellers: A randomized, double-blind placebo-controlled clinical trial. Nutrients,8(4), 182. https://doi.org/10.3390/nu8040182

241   Humphries, S. (2017, October 17). Sodium ascorbate/ vitamin C treatment of whooping cough. Retrieved from http://drsuzanne.net/2017/10/sodium-ascorbate-vitamin-c-treatment-of-whooping-cough-suzanne-humphries-md/

242   Zacharioudakis, I. M., Zervou, F. N., Ziakas, P. D., & Mylonakis, E. (2014). Meta-analysis of methicillin-resistant staphylococcus aureus colonization and risk of infection in dialysis patients. Journal of the American Society of Nephrology,25(9), 2131-2141. https://doi.org/10.1681/asn.2013091028

243   Wallock-Richards, D., Doherty, C. J., Doherty, L., Clarke, D. J., Place, M., Govan, J. R., & Campopiano, D. J. (2014). Garlic revisited: Antimicrobial activity of allicin-containing garlic extracts against burkholderia cepacia complex. PLoS ONE,9(12). https://doi.org/10.1371/journal.pone.0112726

244   Chang, J. S., Wang, K. C., Yeh, C. F., Shieh, D. E., & Chiang, L. C. (2013). Fresh ginger (Zingiber officinale) has anti-viral activity against human respiratory syncytial virus in human respiratory tract cell lines. Journal of Ethnopharmacology,145(1), 146-151. https://doi.org/10.1016/j.jep.2012.10.043

245   Hewlings, S., & Kalman, D. (2017). Curcumin: A review of its effects on human health. Foods MDPI,6(10), 92. https://doi.org/10.3390/foods6100092

246   Acharya, N., Penukonda, S., Shcheglova, T., Hagymasi, A. T., Basu, S., & Srivastava, P. K. (2017). Endocannabinoid system acts as a regulator of immune homeostasis in the gut. Proceedings of the National Academy of Sciences,114(19), 5005-5010. https://doi/10.1073/pnas.1612177114

247   Pandey, R., Mousawy, K., Nagarkatti, M., & Nagarkatti, P. (2009). Endocannabinoids and immune regulation. Pharmacological Research,60(2), 85-92. https://doi.org/10.1016/j.phrs.2009.03.019

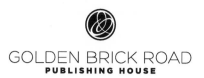

GOLDEN BRICK ROAD
PUBLISHING HOUSE

Link arms with us as we pave new paths to a better and more expansive world.

Golden Brick Road Publishing House (GBRPH) is a small, independently initiated boutique press created to provide social-innovation entrepreneurs, experts, and leaders a space in which they can develop their writing skills and content to reach existing audiences as well as new readers.

Serving an ambitious catalogue of books by individual authors, GBRPH also boasts a unique co-author program that capitalizes on the concept of "many hands make light work." GBRPH works with our authors as partners. Thanks to the value, originality, and fresh ideas we provide our readers, GBRPH books are now available in bookstores across North America.

We aim to develop content that effects positive social change while empowering and educating our members to help them strengthen themselves and the services they provide to their clients.

Iconoclastic, ambitious, and set to enable social innovation, GBRPH is helping our writers/partners make cultural change one book at a time.

Inquire today at www.goldenbrickroad.pub

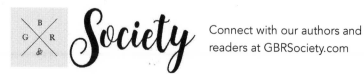

Connect with our authors and readers at GBRSociety.com